Blood, Guts and Tears

Blood, Guts and Tears

True Stories of Courage

by

Brent Braunworth

Pittsburgh, PA

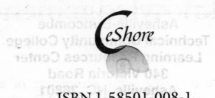

ISBN 1-58501-008-1

Trade Paperback
© Copyright 1999 Brent Braunworth
All rights reserved
First Printing—2000
Library of Congress #98-88535

Request for information should be addressed to:

CeShore Publishing Company
The Sterling Building
440 Friday Road
Pittsburgh, PA 15209
www.ceshore.com

Cover design: Michelle Vennare - SterlingHouse Publisher
Typesetting: Drawing Board Studios
CeShore is an imprint of SterlingHouse Publisher, Inc.

Printed in Canada

Acknowledgements

In an attempt to make some semblance of a dedication here, I must emulate one of my favorite "Thank you's" of all time.

First I dedicate this book to God, without whom I am nothing. Although I know He and I have not always seen eye to eye and my concentration is rarely on what it should be, I feel I make an admirable attempt to do His good through my job.

Next I want to thank my family, especially Mary, Cory and Christina, for putting up with my mood swings, my careers and my other crap. This includes both the Braunworth and Jackson clans.

I also want to thank my real friends, who are becoming less and less each year, but who are nonetheless too numerous to list here.

Lastly I want to thank the firefighter, the average Joe, who may or may not be in charge of an engine or a rescue truck, but works hard, and tries to live the American Dream by raising a family. He doesn't have an inflated ego or a fancy title or consciously seeks any glory whatsoever.

He's the real hero.

The Haunting

Sometimes, on lonely nights, I like to sit outside under the stars and let the ghosts of patients I've lied to visit me...

* * *

The call that usually comes to mind is the time (and it always starts that way) we were dispatched to a "car versus tree" somewhere in the south end of town.

Although I can't now recall which street it was, I remember the night and the scene vividly.

It had been a busy night on the rescue truck. I'd had maybe 45 minutes of sleep, having gone on two assaults and an SOB (shortness of breath)- all after midnight.

We arrived at the dark, winding, little road to find an eerie kind of peace. It was all so quiet I figured it was a false alarm at first. Our headlights were the only flicker of life that shone on the street and we were soon at its end.

Swearing under my breath I told my driver "Turn around; maybe we missed it." Sure enough, in a field right by the entrance to the road was a car straddling a palm tree, it fronds blowing easily in the wind.

"My God!" said my driver after seeing the damage. The entire front end of the vehicle seemed to be obliterated by the king-size palm which had probably stood there for 50 years.

I told my second medic to get the gear and I rushed to the car, thinking this would probably be another DOA.

He was seventeen, I figured—his chest pressed securely against the steering column; his head, having shattered the windshield, was leaning between the top of the steering wheel and the shattered glass. Bits and pieces of clotted blood were scattered everywhere.

Stabilizing his neck, I felt for a pulse.

"Oh God," said a squeaky voice. "My dad's gonna kill me."

Shocked that the kid was still alive, I said, "Relax- we'll have ya outa here in a minute. You're gonna be fine."

That was the first lie. He would *not* be fine and I knew that.

I yelled for a c-collar and for my partner to call for the engine company and contact the hospital to let them know what we had. I knew we'd have trouble getting the kid out of the car by ourselves.

From what I could see it seemed his legs were crumpled under the dashboard, but the rest of his body was basically free.

"Where do ya hurt?" I asked.

"My legs....my arms....my chest," he said, then began to cry. "It was the first time I took the RX-7 out....I only had two beers....My dad's gonna kill me..."

My driver was cranking up the Jaws of Life already and my partner was helping me put on the collar. The PD and a tow truck had just arrived.

"What's your name?" I asked while slipping an 02 mask on him.

"Kenny," he muttered through the mask.

"Just stay cool, Kenny. You'll be all right- we're gonna get ya outa here in just a minute."

I told my partner to start an IV line of Ringers in his left arm as the right was obviously fractured.

As he finished a quick secondary survey, he looked up and said, "No seatbelt. He looks as if he hit the steering wheel pretty hard. His belly seems kinda rigid, too. Maybe he's guarding, I dunno. I also think I have decreased lung sounds on the right."

"Kenny," I said. "Are you breathing all right?"

"Yeah, I guess. It's hard to breathe sometimes." He didn't appear to be having any difficulty.

The engine company arrived. My driver had already started clipping the "A" posts of the car so we could peel back the roof and place the kid on a backboard, taking him out the top.

I directed my partner to tell the company what to do and he placed a blanket over me and Kenny so we wouldn't get cut up by any glass.

Kenny's pulse rate was 130 and his blood pressure was 90/50. I knew we just had a few minutes.

"You're gonna be all right, kid," I said. "Just hold on....You go to school around here?"

"Yeah."

"You play football?"

"Yeah."

"Good. It builds character and makes ya tough," I said. Under the blanket I could hear the continuous buzzing of the Jaws cutting up the car. Every once in a while the car would jump which meant something else had been accomplished and we were closer to our goal. Kenny was silent and I sat behind him in the backseat with my hands holding his neck, praying for time. It was like we were the only two people on Earth.

My partner had gotten the IV and we were running in as much fluid as we could.

It took the company just a few more seconds to finish slicing up the car and peel back the roof.

"Okay kid, we're gonna slide you out," I said.

With everyone's help, we attempted to pick Kenny up and slid him on a backboard.

"My legs, my legs!" he cried.

"There's too much of him under the dash, Brent,"

somebody yelled over the buzzing. "We're gonna hafta use the chains to lift the steering column and raise the dashboard."

"Okay," I said. "Make it quick." Then I turned back to Kenny. "How do ya feel, kid?"

"Not so good." Even with the limited light we had, he seemed to be getting paler.

"Kenny," I said. "I wanna help ya, but you gotta help me. I gotta put another needle in the side of your neck to give you more fluid, okay?"

He nodded as best he could, beginning to cry again. "I don't wanna die," he said.

"Listen to me," I answered back, my nose inches from his face. "You're gonna be just fine. You're not gonna die, believe me."

I had one of the firefighters hold traction on his neck while I removed the collar and slid a 14 gauge IV catheter into his left external jugular vein. It was good that I got the line, but it wasn't so good that he let me do it so easily.

That meant his pressure was dropping.

At least we now had two bags of Ringers flowing in him to replace all the blood he'd lost internally.

With the aid of the Jaws of Life my firefighters began to raise the steering column and the dashboard. We were working as fast as we could and I was hoping we'd have enough time.

"Okay, Brent," said the Captain. "We're ready to move him."

"Ken," I said. "We're gonna get ya out. Relax, but ya gotta promise me you'll wear your seatbelt from now on."

Kenny's head kind of slumped back in my hands. I watched his eyes quickly dilate. "He's coded," I yelled, feeling for a pulse. "Let's get him out now!"

Again we attempted to slide what was now a lifeless Kenny out onto a board. "Brent," said my partner, still yelling above the continuous buzz of the Jaws. "He won't go. His foot is lodged outside from a hole in the floor, between the bottom of the car and the ground."

"Pull on it!" I yelled. "We need to get him going now."

"He won't go, Brent."

"He's got to! Yank on it!"

We pulled and yanked, but the RX-7 wouldn't relinquish its hold on Kenny. I even had them put the airbags under the car to elevate it, but still his leg was caught.

We attempted to decompress the right side of Kenny's chest with a needle in order to release the air which had been building up there because of a ruptured lung, but for some reason, it didn't work.

"I dunno," said my partner. "I dunno what's wrong."

"All right, forget it. We need to start compressions."

"We can't; he's still too close to the dash. I can't get positioned."

"We need to get him out *now*. Keep working," I yelled back.

We had been handling the scene so calmly before and now it was becoming nothing short of chaotic.

Dripping with sweat, I attempted to intubate him (place a tube down his trachea) and that's when the Captain finally put his hand on my shoulder.

"Brent," he said calmly. "We've been here for 20 minutes. We can't get him out...It's over."

"No, no, just another minute. We can get–" I looked around at the faces who'd helped me. They were looking at me as if I was some kind of Captain Bligh who didn't know when to give up his ship.

I stopped ventilating the kid and slowly got out of the car. "Cover him," I said.

"Hey – ya did all ya could," somebody else added.

I called the hospital back on the radio to tell them what had happened and that I had called an approximately seventeen-year-old male at 0437 hours. After that I contacted my medical director for a rubber-stamp approval.

"My dad's gonna kill me." His voice still rang in my head.

We began packing up our gear, trying to find all the

scattered equipment. Once the Jaws had been silenced, that eerie peace returned.

It was over- nothing else could be done.

Eyes darted over at me from time to time and whispers of what we could have done or what we should have done were now the background noise. A few people from the houses down the street had gathered to see what all the commotion was.

They shook their heads; they seemed to glance over at me and then down at the ground.

A lot of things crossed my mind: things like a seventeen-year-old taking his dad's car for a spin for the first time, a father receiving a visit from a sheriff and finding out his son was now dead and finally how I felt about it.

I looked over at Kenny's now uncovered, lifeless body: tubes and needles still intact and violating him.

Seventeen-years-old. What a waste. He should be parked by the beach somewhere with a girl learning about sex, not getting ready to be put in a body bag. It just wasn't fair.

Sitting down on the back of the truck, I felt the sting and the cold of the foul night air against my face. Air that reeked of drunken teens, errors of judgment and tired firefighters and paramedics who tried to keep pace.

I put my head in my hands. Everyday people were always the first to criticize, but when they needed help who did they call?

It wasn't my kid- why should it bother me so much? *Hell, there would be Kennys all across the world who'd die tonight*, I thought.

I looked at the cigarette in my hand and I had to laugh. I thought I'd quit. Life's problems seem comparatively minimal when you've seen children die. And I laughed hysterically for a minute until I felt the tears well up in my eyes and I sobbed silently.

So sometimes on lonely nights I like to sit outside under the stars and let the ghosts of patients I lied to visit me: those with symptomatic chest pains whom I told would be all right, victims of shootings and stabbings I swore would live.

And sometimes I hear a squeaky voice say, "My dad's gonna kill me."

I turn and no one's there. Then I think about a father sitting alone and solemn because his son was gone and he's just realized he's missed the best years of his life and I wonder who's responsible.

SWAT Boy

"Just another hostage situation." That's what seemed to be the attitude of most of the other guys. But for me and my partner David Nelson, this being our first, it was strange at best. Any minute we would be running into an apartment of a man who was holding a knife to his girlfriend's throat and there was no way of telling what would happen.

Over his black mask I could see that David's eyes were filled with boyish anticipation, whereas mine, I'm sure, were reflecting the fact that I had a healthy respect for this type of situation.

Dressed in all black, complete with a heavy bulletproof vest and ballistic helmet, I crouched low by the stairwell, waiting for the signal to move to the second floor. As I did this, I pondered how it was that I, a West Palm Beach Firefighter-paramedic, came to be in this situation.

My partner and I are known as SWAT-medics, more or less a cross between a paramedic and a tactically trained SWAT police officer.

* * *

The word comes to me from dispatch. I am the downtown supervisor that day, stepping up from my regular paramedic Lieutenant spot to EMS Captain, whose responsibility is to supervise all the shift fire-medics as well as all the emergency medical calls.

"Braunworth," I mutter into the receiver. It's now 2330 hours and I've had a very busy day.

"Yeah, Captain, we got an incident in the north end of

town and sir, since you're a SWAT-medic we were told to put you on alert."

"What is it?"

"It's a guy holding his girlfriend hostage with a knife to her throat."

I tell the Battalion Chief, the "fire suppression end" Supervisor who runs the shift, and he is not happy either. He doesn't want to lose one of his men to a PD call; plus, he doesn't want the responsibility.

* * *

Placing highly trained medical personnel with law enforcement tactical entry teams, better known as SWAT teams, is not a new concept at all. Historically, it can be traced back to the military in which SEAL teams and other individualized units began requiring someone be trained with advanced medical knowledge since hospitals were usually large distances away.

More recently fire and police departments have begun to recognize the importance of this specialized job and cities like Miami, Florida have been collaborating in this area for the last fifteen years.

The SWAT-medic program first came to my attention in the form of a notice indicating that tryouts for the West Palm Police Department SWAT Team would be held in the month of March 1990.

To qualify, one had to pass two days of physical and mental tests, including a 3 mile jog in thirty minutes and a 1.5 mile run in twelve minutes. There was also a 100-hundred-yard man-carry, a 20 foot rope climb and an eight foot wall to scale.

That didn't sound too strenuous to me. At age twenty-nine, I was in pretty good shape, so I thought. In those two days I must have done 500 push-ups and run 15 miles.

Six of us fire-medics tried out; three would actually finish the two days and only two would make the team.

* * *

I leave the central fire station and go up to the scene to see what is exactly going on. Maybe it's not so bad, I think. I still have a lot of paperwork to do.

Two city blocks are roped off and you can see both patrolmen and detectives scurry about the darkened scene.

I am in no position to see it, but there is a man who's shouting outside a second story apartment. He yells that he wants to be left alone and he won't give up. I gather this is the guy. (I later find out that he had his girlfriend in a choke hold with a knife to her neck the entire time he was speaking).

My Battalion Chief and a rescue unit are by my truck when I get back. I explain the situation and about that time I get a call from dispatch on the radio saying that the SWAT team is officially calling me out.

* * *

SWAT teams are normally utilized when a situation arises that is above and beyond the normally trained and equipped police officer's capability. Certain situations can require the use of specialized weapons and tactics. High-risk search warrants, hostage situations and barricaded suspects are thought to these types of situations.

The most common SWAT mission, by far, is the search warrant. Most warrants are drug related, but because crack dealers can afford a lot of security, most of them are considered "high-risk." Many of these so-called "businessmen" have more firepower and advanced weapons than the Tactical teams which serve the warrants.

SWAT-medics, dressed in black from the tip of their ballistic helmet to their black fatigues and boots, look exactly like other SWAT officers except they carry a 20 pound backpack. In the heavy backpacks are all the necessary medical and trauma gear needed to initiate emergency care in a hostile environment, minutes before a fire rescue truck would even be dispatched to a scene.

* * *

About 30 minutes after I am notified about the "Call out", I am told by a patrol Sergeant to wait by my truck which is blocking off Dixie Highway with two other patrol cars.

Within minutes I see the indistinguishable, white SWAT van pull up. The doors open up, but it is dark inside. I hop in the back and am whisked away; the whole process is slick and unassuming, taking less than 15 seconds. If you weren't paying attention you might've thought I'd just vanished.

* * *

The lights go on and I see eight other SWAT officers sitting on the benches. The Sergeant points to my SWAT bag. "Better get ready," he says. "We'll be there in a minute and briefed in less than five."

The average "call-out" happens once a week, normally on a day when search warrants have built up and the police department supervisors decide to do them all in one outing. Oh, sure, we get called out many times for dangerous drug deals with only an hour's notice, but that doesn't usually happen more than once a month.

For a typical search warrant there are usually seven SWAT officers, including the two medics. During a "briefing", all are given specific assignments on the entry team. The medics, since they are trained exactly like the other officers, are usually given another role in addition to their normal medical one.

The entry team is made up of two *door men* who have the responsibility of getting the team into the house.

The two *cover men* usually carry the automatic machine guns in order to protect the *door men* and then have the added responsibility of entering the house first. Their job is to stop any initial threat and get to the back of the house as quickly as possible.

The *Team Leader*, usually a Sergeant, carries the shotgun, as well as the tear gas or "heavy-duty" pepper spray. He enters after the door men in order to direct the team in the event problems are encountered or the situation suddenly changes.

The SWAT-medic (or medics) enter last, securing any "downed" suspects and, of course, treating any injuries if necessary.

One learns on this team to complete one task at a time and do it well. Others are depending on you; their lives can depend on your actions. That is the epitome of a TEAM.

A SWAT teams' best tactic is the element of surprise. Within seconds we appear out of nowhere like raiders in black, all with guns drawn and aimed, swarming out of the darkness so quickly and efficiently our victims don't know what's going on until it's too late.

* * *

Concealed by trees and hedges, we are addressed by Captain Bruce, our SWAT Commander, and Team Leader, Sergeant Sowers. The "bad-guy" is a Hispanic drug user who has taken his girlfriend hostage for approximately two hours. Neighbors of the apartment complex called 911 and all others in the building have been evacuated.

The suspect is holding a large kitchen knife to his girlfriend's throat. Initial sightings reported that there might be blood on the walls inside the apartment. It is a two bed-room apartment and the blinds are drawn; there is only one direction to enter or depart the house, specifically through either the front door or front windows. It is unknown if there are other weapons in the house.

Negotiators had the suspect on the phone prior to our arrival. He wanted to be left alone. Tactics are discussed.

I am almost dressed, complete with my tactical entry vest that extends from my neck to my groin. I finish by placing my nomex mask over my face underneath my helmet.

Assignments are given. Captain Bruce grabs me and David. "You two will be the last inside, behind me. There could be injuries, so stay on your toes," he adds.

Bruce's radio squawks and he turns to the team. "We have him back on the phone and he wants to come out and talk with one of the negotiators," he says.

With that little notice we converge on the building, each of us knowing our role. The problem is we don't know if he'll come out with or without his girlfriend.

In seconds we are at the building. The first few entry of-ficers are low crawling under windows to get on either side of the apartment. David, myself and Captain Bruce are on the stairwell awaiting direction from Sergeant Sowers upstairs.

We are on these same stairs for what seems like an eternity. The thought goes through my mind that maybe something's happening and we were forgotten. It's a warm night and sweat begins to roll into my eyes.

Finally we are told to move to the second floor. I take a kneeling position in a doorway three apartments from the suspect's.

Minutes pass. I reposition my handgun in my fingers and rest my arm from pointing on my knee. Not a sound can be heard. I notice occasional movement by those who surround the door; it is indiscernible to anyone except for us. We are all in doorways, around corners, under windows, either kneeling or on our bellies.

A curtain is slightly drawn in the apartment. He is looking outside, expecting a trap. I hear Captain Bruce mutter into his radio something about having the negotiator tell him he's outside and down the corridor.

The door is cracked and slowly begins to open. Light falls on the balcony for the first time from the apartment. Like roaches we move back into the darkness. He's got the girl with him- knife at her throat. He looks down the corridor and that's when we pounce. Our first man comes from behind the door grabbing the knife; another separates the girl from him and ties up his other hand. We swarm on him like South Florida mosquitoes at dusk. I join in and jump on the pile finding it is difficult to wrestle on a three foot wide balcony.

In less than a minute he is subdued and cuffed. I break free from the pile and move into the apartment following the girl. David and others are helping to get the suspect to his feet. I find her walking around nervously and have to convince her to sit on the couch. Looking around I notice the blood on the walls is actually red paint.

She seems exhausted, crying. "Are you hurt?" I ask speaking through my mask.

"No, I'm okay. He didn't cut me."

I take my mask and helmet off to examine her. Other SWAT officers run around us, checking the apartment making sure it's safe. As I reach to take a pulse rate from her wrist, she gently pulls away.

"It's okay," I say. "I'm a paramedic, too. I wanna make sure you're all right."

She looks at me as if I'm crazy, but gives me her wrist.

* * *

The first question always posed to me is how it makes me feel to be both a paramedic and a SWAT officer. I consider myself a lifesaver first and everything else is second. That's why I was picked for this team anyway, certainly not for my legal knowledge. I take it as an extension of the fire department, but it is a conflicting duality. As a fire-medic, people like to see you; when you're called to the scene, you are welcomed as someone who is friendly and helpful. As a police officer, you're not always wanted, because if you're there, it usually means someone is going to jail.

To date, David and I have completed over 140 SWAT missions. We have had 20 injuries ranging anywhere from lacerated arms to heat exhaustion, to pregnant suspects about to give birth, and still the most common question asked is how I am affected by it.

I am writing out bills only half-watching TV with my son, who is four. "Dad," he says, "Is that what you do?"

I look up at the TV. It's one of those emergency 911 shows and they have tape from an actual SWAT hostage situation. Someone with an over-dramatic, theatrical voice is narrating.

The hostages are lined up in front of a store while a gun-toting bad guy in a ski-mask walks back and forth. The plan is for a sniper to "take out" this guy and then the other members of the SWAT team will rush in from behind.

I watch intently as the sniper misses his shot and the bad guy begins shooting the hostages at random. The SWAT team races in and he is killed - four or five dead.

"Dad, Dad, Dad..."

"Huh?" I reply still mesmerized. "It's just a movie; it's not real," I say automatically, changing the channel with the remote.

"No, Dad. Lemme ask you sumthin'. Is that what you do?"

"Yeah. Sometimes."

"Could that happen to you?"

"No," I say smiling. "Daddy is too mean and ornery. Besides, it's not real- it's just a movie."

He looks at the TV and then back at me. And I wonder if he knows I'm sweating profusely.

A Long Day's Night

Crazy can be a word used to describe the "insane", the "mentally deranged", or any night when you're working as a fire-medic in the city of West Palm.

I believe it was a Monday. I was working on a ALS (Advanced Life Support) engine, a relatively new feature of the West Palm Beach Fire Department which places seasoned fire-medics, who work normally on the smaller, ambulance-like fire rescue trucks, on pumpers to provide a quicker, more advanced response to the sick and injured.

The days on trucks like these were somewhat more complex but usually not as bustling as their smaller sister truck. That's what I thought, but as usual I was wrong.

The day started off somewhat slow with a formalized review of hazardous materials response put on by our training division to ensure state guidelines. This type of call, like the ALS Engine I was on that day, was more or less a new responsibility added to our potpourri of duties. We've always responded to these types of emergencies -hell, we're the fire department- but it was only recently that the Federal government came up with rules and regulations on how we should handle them.

Well, that's how we spent our morning, attending a refresher class, reviewing what would probably change in the next few years. We grabbed a quick lunch and then the calls began.

In most cities a call for an assault at 12:30 on a Monday afternoon might seem odd, but it's par for the course in

West Palm Beach, Florida and no one is ever really surprised whenever a call like this comes in.

When we got there we found it was not an assault at all, but a drunken man on a bike who ran into not one road sign but two and then the center of a telephone pole before he abruptly stopped. It was at that point, I'm sure, that some good Samaritan passerby with a cellular phone had called 911.

He tried to tell us in South American English that he had been assaulted, but we could tell by the gashes on his head and the bloodied signs and pole that that just wasn't so.

This is just another part of being a fire-medic, deciphering the truth from the lies. It's amazing how many times a patient will lie to you because you look like the police or they just don't trust anyone in a uniform.

We cleaned the patient up and advised him he needed to be checked at an ER. He refused in perfectly good English and bid us farewell leaving his now-broken bike in the street deciding that it would be best to stagger the rest of the way home, wherever that may have been. I figured he was just a busy guy with a lot more drinking to do. Hell, it was only 12:45 p.m.

The clouds began to look ominous as we packed up our gear. The first crack of lightning happened when I got in the front seat of the cab and a moment later we were dispatched to a fire alarm in our area.

We knew it probably wouldn't be anything but an electrical surge, but we stopped the truck anyway and fought putting on our fire garb in the rain and subsequently, raced to the address. It was indeed a false alarm and for the next two hours we chased false alarms from one end of the city to the other.

In the middle of all that we responded to a well-known crack-addict residence for a possible poisoning. At first, whoever called wouldn't open the door because he didn't believe we were the Fire Department, not even after seeing the fire engine or even our badges. Finally he gave in and we were allowed to enter.

The young man had smoked something he thought was crack and now had a burning sensation in his throat. We checked him out, started an IV and sent him up to Good Sam Hospital with one of our rescue trucks. He was really confused once three other guys showed with a stretcher.

The time was 3:05 p.m. We got back to the station in just enough time so that we could back the truck into the bay and shut the automatic garage door before we got our next call.

The most common medical alarm in the beginning or at the end of a rainstorm is always an auto accident. You can usually count on going to at least one in your area whenever it rains- and you know how much it rains in South Florida.

It was a car versus a truck head-on, but at a low MPH with moderate damage. Two woman drivers. They were more upset then anything, having maybe a few cuts. Both had been wearing their seat belts and it could have been a lot worse if they hadn't. One began to complain later of neck pain, so we immobilized her to a long spine board with a c-collar and, since she was stable, sent her up to Good Sam on a local ambulance. If she hadn't been very stable we would have called for one of the fire department's own rescue trucks for transport.

We cleared that scene and were immediately beeped out to another auto accident out of our area. The city was going crazy. After a few minutes, we got there and found no accident; by now it was raining like hell.

I got on the radio and back we went to our own zone for more of the same. A rescue truck was already there when we arrived, so we took direction and helped them extricate the patients from the car and ready them for transport.

It was a pretty bad wreck with two serious injuries, one older man with chest pain who hit the steering wheel and his wife who had numbness in her right arm.

We loaded them up in the rescue truck with the other

fire-medics and they went merrily on their way to West Palm's own trauma center, St. Mary's Hospital.

We stayed at the scene in the rain, getting soaked to the bone, securing the cars and waiting for both PD and a wrecker to arrive.

We got back at the station at about 5:30 p.m. and started to talk about what might be for dinner. Normally most of the guys cook, but no one had brought anything in that day. We decided on picking something up at a local fish restaurant to make it easy on ourselves.

Our food would be ready in about an hour, so I sat down to try to begin the voluminous amount of paperwork needed for each and every call. To say what I had to do required multiple duplication would be an understatement: we seem to have to document everything about three or four times, but in a paramilitary organization you don't question orders- you follow them. That's one of the reasons why these types of problems are never corrected.

I was into my paperwork about fifteen minutes when the next call came across the speakers. I could hear my guys groan as they walked ploddingly to the truck.

He was about 6' 2" with long scraggly hair and an even more unruly beard. Standing on the street corner when we arrived, he was spouting off Biblical verses and political rhetoric interchangeably. It had stopped raining.

I peeled myself out of my seat and ambled over to where he stood. "What seems to be the problem?" I asked.

Immediately I was sorry I asked since I was then bombarded with verbal propaganda. "What's the problem?" he mimicked, raising his arms. "The human race- that's the problem. Humanity is the most self-serving-"

My medic partner wearily began to take the patient's vital signs, but the man jerked away and my partner was promptly dubbed a "heathen."

All of the sudden, he was leaning over me saying things like, "Agent Orange. That mean anything to you?"

Looking behind himself to and fro, he moved in closer.

"I'm a former Green Beret, Delta force, Navy Seal- know what I mean?" He breathed heavily, looking for my response. His breath could have suffocated a small animal.

I shrugged. "I thought you usually were in one or the other of those kinds of units, not all three at once."

He turned in disgust saying we would all be damned by God.

"Look, are you hurt? Have you taken any drugs?" asked my partner.

"No," he said, "and I'm not going to talk to you." He folded his arms which were covered with the sleeves of a raggedy green jacket. I gathered it was military issue or at least he wanted us to think that.

It took the police department another ten minutes to get there. I told the officer that this gentleman didn't appear to be injured and that I thought perhaps the best thing for him would be a little counseling at County Mental Health. There wasn't much we could do for him.

He nodded, somewhat irritated since I had just dropped the ball in his court. "Okay," he said.

The big man resisted only slightly as we escorted him into the back of the PD unit. He looked into my eyes. "What do see when you turn off the lights?" he asked.

I didn't reply as I didn't know if it was a threat or not. My partner came over and whispered in my ear as our driver began to load up our equipment. "Don't worry," he said, "but you just put John the Baptist in a mental institution."

"Could've been worse." I added, "it could've been Jesus Christ, Himself. We'd all go to hell."

"Can't be any worse then Rescue 1 on a Friday night."

The time was now 7:00 p.m. We were en route to pick up our dinner, more or less discussing the day's events when the next one came in.

We got to the address given in three minutes. Outside on the sidewalk was a crowd of people. With the sun having set and no working street lights, it was hard to see whether there was someone in the crowd with a problem or it was your everyday West Palm gathering. I grabbed the "OB kit" and the "trauma bag" out of the compartment since the reference dispatched over the radio had been a woman in labor.

In the middle of the crowd there was a Haitian woman, approximately thirty years-old whom we surmised was the patient. She looked to be the only one who was pregnant. We asked questions, but since none of them spoke English we basically got nothing that could help us. My Haitian leaves much to be desired even on a good day.

We couldn't pinpoint what was wrong, only that she was in some sort of pain. I advised dispatch that I needed a Haitian-speaking police officer and she advised back that PD was all tied up.

Finally an elderly woman stepped forward and with broken English said she might be able to help, stating something about being "biannual." I didn't know what that meant, but soon she was conversing with the patient, who was now seated in a chair on the sidewalk which we requested and somehow received, while I took vital signs.

The woman who was translating came back with all the right answers: the patient was not term yet, this was her first child and her water had not broken. This meant she would not deliver soon and she could probably go by ambulance to the ER and not one of our rescue trucks. I went to the pumper to get away from the noise of the crowd so I could call on the radio for an ambulance while my partner and driver timed the patient's contractions.

Leisurely I walked back from the truck, thinking about a fish sandwich, when I heard my name being yelled. It was my partner. It seemed like this patient who was not going to have this baby anytime soon had, in fact, just delivered. I stumbled over to him in the darkness, fumbling with my flashlight and the OB kit. There sat a full-sized baby in my partner's gloved hands with this strange looking greenish-brown jelly all over everything.

"He's not breathing," said my partner.

"That's meconium staining," I added. This was the

worst case scenario for a newborn: when a baby is born, if he becomes stressed during the delivery, he may defecate. If this mixes with the amniotic fluid and is inhaled into the baby's mouth, then, because of its thickness, it can and usually will compromise the baby's airway. In other words, this was not good and we had to work fast.

We started chest compressions, since there was also no pulse, and I began to get ready to suction the baby's mouth. This was key to any successful resuscitation of a newborn like this- you had to get the meconium out from blocking the baby's trachea.

Along the way I canceled the ambulance and told dispatch I needed a rescue truck ASAP. Once I completed suctioning, I figured I'd need to intubate the child (put a tube down his trachea).

Just as I positioned myself to begin suctioning and as my driver was getting ready to cut the cord, my flashlight went out. It was pitch black; I couldn't see a damn thing. A strange question rang through my head: "What do you see when you turn off the lights?"

The answer was FEAR.

"Get me a #$%#$% light!" I screamed. My driver ran back to the truck like a dog after a cat. A moment later I heard him huffing and we again had light.

The cord was cut and I began to suction out the little boy's airway, working gingerly so as not to make the problem worse before it got better, but I still couldn't see well enough. That's when the ambulance pulled up.

There has been so much talk of the private ambulances taking over our jobs that, at first, I really wasn't happy to see them. But I shook that feeling off and yelled that I needed to use the back of their truck.

Sliding out of the front seat, the driver met us by saying, "We were just in the neighborhood-"

I cut him off. "I need light to suction this kid."

He nodded, sprinting with me as I both covered and carried the baby to the back of the ambulance. I found the stretcher and began to work, hoping that we still had time, and suctioned deep in the little boy's mouth using a tube that is normally placed in the trachea, not knowing if this "school technique" would work. My partner was still doing compressions, but paused for a moment. "I dunno what you just did but I can feel a pulse in his chest."

While concentrating, "Huh?" was all I could manage, but I could see his little chest thumping away.

I suctioned a little more in the same manner. My partner reported the baby's pulse was 120 and he was stopping compressions. Just as I went to suction one more time, there was a cry, a breath and then regular breathing with more crying mixed in.

"Oh my God," I said in astonishment. The baby was now moving and coughing, trying to get rid of the rest of the meconium on his own.

Our rescue truck had been there for a few minutes and the other fire-medics had checked out the mom and cleaned up the scene. I turned the baby over to them.

Although I had done the suctioning, everyone else, including my partner, the other fire-medics and even the ambulance crew had offered advice, assistance and finally moral support. I thanked them all. It was amazing: two entities, one public and one private, who always seemed at odds with each another, had worked together, perhaps both of us realizing that this was the kind of thing we were here for.

By the time I got back in my ALS pumper, I was exhausted. The time was 8:45 p.m. and now there were only two of us. Due to budgetary problems, sometimes we ride only two fire-medics on certain rescue trucks on certain days. Subsequently, we had to loan our driver to that truck so he could drive the two fire-medics to Good Samaritan Hospital's ER while they worked on the baby in the back.

"Let's go eat," I said and my partner agreed, smiling. After picking up our dinners, I began to organize my paperwork while I awaited the rescue truck to bring my driver back.

Finally, I settled down to eat. One bite- that's all I got.

A call came in for a man complaining of chest pains in a house on Flagler Drive. We sat down to treat the sixty-eight-year old man, but he bluntly refused any care.

"Why did you call us?" I asked.

"I didn't call you, ya idiot, my daughter did. Now leave me alone."

I tried to reason with the man, explaining that he needed both pre-hospital and in-hospital medical care. He adamantly refused. I shrugged, his daughter shrugged. Legally there was nothing we could do.

On the way back to the station, I found it curious why some people would call 911 demanding care for relatively minor things, like lacerated fingers and twisted ankles, and others, like the last man who had a real complaint, wouldn't accept any help at all.

The time was 11:30 p.m. I had taken two bites from my soggy fish sandwich before I threw it out. I instead had a Diet Coke for dinner.

I began to work on my paperwork. At 1:00 a.m. I took a break. Almost done; maybe another half-hour.

Time: 1:01 a.m. Our next call came in. It was raining again and a repeat of the fire alarm scramble was on. Over the radio I heard one of our rescue trucks going to a shooting in the north end and two pumpers responding to a possible structure fire. I groaned wondering if this night would ever end.

"My kingdom for a shower," I said. My driver didn't get it, but continued to sleepily drive through the rain. This one turned out to be another false alarm.

We got back at the station a little after 2:00 a.m. I took a shower and decided to forget the paperwork until shift change at 7:30. 1 needed sleep and I found it in a recliner in the living room while watching HBO.

The next thing I knew somebody was tugging at my shirt. *Thank God*, I thought, *it's the new crew and I can go home.* Once again, I was wrong. It was my partner, "Brent," he said. "Come on; we got a call." I'd slept through the alarm.

The time was 4:30 a.m. We arrived at a local progressive rock bar for an assault. I couldn't tell if the place was still open or not. PD was there already controlling the scene and one of the officers explained that a riot had nearly broken out. We counted twelve injuries. They seemed all minor in nature, so instead of calling for additional units, we decided to divvy the patients up three ways.

I bandaged up my four, all with minor cuts and bruises from fighting, and sent them on their way by car to the ER. Out of the other eight, only one, a twenty-one-year-old male, was hurt seriously experiencing neck pain after being hit in the face. We placed a c-collar on him and put him on a long spine board. While we waited for the ambulance it began to rain again.

On the way back to the station, we pulled up to a stop sign. My partner banged furiously on the window over my head from his jump seat situated behind me. I turned to see what he wanted.

"Look!" he said motioning to the street. "Look- it's John the Baptist!"

He was hard to miss. Standing on the corner, complete with untamed hair and beard, swinging his green jacket over his head, he pointed his finger at our truck and seemed to be laughing at us.

Our eyes met. *What do you see when you turn off the lights?* my brain repeated the question again.

"I can't believe he's back out here before our shift is even up," my partner wailed. "He's probably had more sleep than us."

"What is it? What is it?" my driver asked, trying to look around me.

"Just a madman laughing in the rain," I said with a yawn.

"Look at him! The guy's a nut," my partner continued.

Our eyes met again and I had to smile. In the last twenty-four hours I had been to over ten assaults, four auto accidents, who knows how many false fire alarms, treated a drunken marathon bicyclist and an incredulous crack-head, talked to a man in denial of his chest pain, and resuscitated one newborn baby in respiratory and cardiac arrest. It was 5:30 in the morning, I was wet, exhausted and hungry and I still had two hours of paperwork to do.

I closed my eyes, counting up all the times I swore I'd quit this job and I wondered who was really crazy.

The Great Garbage Scow Fire

The spark. One devious, little spark caused by something never found: a forgotten cigarette, a hot pipe, a spotlight on a hook dropped on the ground for a second. It started in the conveyer room when garbage was being separated into usable and non-usable. With that piece of trash it moved, via conveyer belt, upwards to the top of the waste plant, some 70 feet above the ground. Along the way, the spark now having turned into full-fledged flames, spewed forth more havoc into the main area trash room.

Life had begun at 1300 degrees Fahrenheit.

Excerpts from Report Engine 6

Engine 6 arrived to find light smoke showing in the area of the Solid Waste Authority and assumed Command. Protective gear was donned and upon further investigation it was found that the entire north complex was filled with smoke. Solid Waste personnel were evacuated and Engine 6 requested additional units at 1923 hours.

Excerpts from Report Engine 5

Engine 5 arrived and was assigned by Command to provide a water source to Engine 6. Engine 5 found two hydrants, one dry. A 5 inch supply line was laid to Engine 6 from the one good hydrant on the SW corner after cutting the back gates and fence to allow for the entry of the pumper and delivery of the line.

The flames at the top of the complex, dropped off by the belt, had grown hungry, exhausting much of the fuel provided it. So fiery arms were tapered back. Unable to feed itself, it smoked and waited, biding its time.

The second set of flames found an overabundance of fuel, in the main trash room, of the kind it liked: paper products, plastics and wood. It was overwhelmed at first, grabbing at everything wet and dry alike. After having trouble organizing, it decided to sit back and smolder and plan.

Lastly, the fire on the conveyer belt, having wasted most of its fuel, chewed on the belt itself. Amiss of any actually flame, it filled the top of the complex with thick, black, toxic smoke, as it tried to survive, weakening the already slack rubber.

* * *

A total of seven units arrived to attempt to bring the fire under control—four pumpers and three rescue trucks. Firefighters were strewn from one end of the complex to the other.

"Rescue 5 arriving at level one staging," I yawned into the mike. Another red-letter day in West Palm Beach. A couple of chest pains, one assault, two auto accidents and now, as dinner was being contemplated, a working fire.

"Rescue 5, report to command in person."

We put on our bunker pants and boots and lugged all of our gear, including air packs, over to the command post walking like sleepy, hesitant children the first day of school.

After a lot of x's and o's on a grease board, I was informed I was going to lead a task force to the top of the Solid Waste plant in order to find out the whereabouts of the fire or fires and possibly extinguish them.

The Commander was an overzealous, little, balding Captain whom had some experience at fires, but was certainly more adept at memos than he was at emergencies. This was comforting since he was sending me into this hellhole. I asked a few pertinent questions about blueprints and conditions and this raised more questions with no answers, unfortunately, and finally I was told my task force was ready.

I figured *what the hell.* It didn't look that bad anyway; besides, it was just a bunch of garbage surrounded by a four walls of 1/4" aluminum siding- a great, big garbage dump. So what if it was 20,000 square feet? How hard could it be? Engine 6 had already cut into one part of the building on the northwest side and found a conveyer belt on fire. How much fire could there be?

Although I was against it, in lieu of blueprints, we were told to take a Solid Waste Foreman with us who knew the intricacies of the building. He had some industrial firefighting experience so we gave him an air pack and headed up the rickety, metal catwalk which spiraled up 70 feet, leading to a variety of work and processing stations.

It was hard to communicate with one another because ofthe smoke and our air masks and the fact there was only room for us to go up single file. Seven of us, all in a row carrying hose and axes, started upward, grabbing the side rails with our gloves, our awkward rubber boots tripping on the metal stairs as the ground slipped further and further away.

About 30 feet up we hooked into the standpipe, the building's water system, required by fire code for any building over 40 feet. With the pumpers down below, they would be able to push the hydranted water up through the pipes of the building so that we could use our hoses to extinguish the fire. Simple, right? That was if the standpipe was working correctly ...and it wasn't.

So, with some us of already low on air after fudging with the system for fifteen minutes, we traipsed back down to the ground so we could change our airpacks and then hump an already charged, attack line onto our backs carrying it back up the catwalk.

The Solid Waste Foreman had been very excited about our progress. "We'll get up there this time," he said, smiling. "I think it's gotta be at the top."

I smiled back good-naturedly. Yeah, we'd get up there

all right, eventually. Why? We should just let it burn anyway, I mused.

The fire in the main trash room was now organized, burning fuel at a steady pace. Flames lept high and it ignored everything, reveling in all its heated glory.

Stumbling in the darkness, we soon found that the hand-rails were somewhat elusive. Sometimes we'd have two, other times none, but mostly we had one to our left, going up. When our pointman found there were none, he'd signal me and we'd each grab hold of our coats, shuffling along like a conga line in the dark, hoping whoever was in front of us didn't fall or we all would.

Every once in a while one of us would slip and the rest of us would snatch a handful of coat and straighten him back up like a Saturday night drunk.

Since the foreman swore he knew all the twists and turns of the cat walk I quickly decided that he should probably lead the way.

Two others followed him, then Duncan Harman and then me. Three newer guys brought up the rear; I wasn't even sure of their names. They were the ones stuck carrying the half-filled fire hose on their backs.

After about 40 feet we were able to begin to see where we were stepping again. This was comforting to me since I was certain I would eventually fall off this monstrosity into a 100 foot pile of garbage only to be separated into usable and non-usable trash the following day.

The foreman motioned that we were going to turn right. Through his mask I heard something muddled about the main trash area. I could hear the roar of what I guessed was machinery as we entered atop the room and soon the roar was deafening. My question was that I thought they had cut all the power to the building to avoid more sparking. We made another right. The flames were ripping up through the catwalk almost to the top of the complex.

The foreman stopped dead in his tracks, causing us to jam up into one another. The flames were licking at our boots; the catwalk creaked with the heat. The foreman and my first man had fallen over each other, arms and legs tangled together. I tried to grab the hose and called on the radio for the engineer to pump more pressure. Boots slipped on the sagging catwalk. The new guys cowered trying to open the nozzle. My hands searched for a handrail and Duncan grabbed my collar to keep me from falling.

The hose was now spewing about half the amount of water it could. "More pressure, more pressure!" I yelled into the mic. It was just enough water to keep us from frying. I heard some garbled reply from the Commander. I pushed my face out the side of my mask to speak more clearly. "This is Task Force 1. I need more water pressure—*now*!"

I felt the hose harden in my free hand. "Open it all the way!" I yelled.

Duncan was reaching over to get some handle on the hoseline and help control it. It was now wiggling around like a snake. "This is Task Force 1- not so much pressure!" I hollered back into the radio, my face free again, the air from my airpack flowing free and uninhibited into the smoky atmosphere.

The hose stopped moving so much. We had it in a full, wide-out fog pattern over our heads. Suddenly, the catwalk seemed to stabilize and stop moving. The heat lessened. Now the foreman and my first man could stand as the roaring had ceased.

I looked around. All that was left was a few moderate looking spot fires. We hit them with straight streams and they would spark up on occasion, but they were basically out. There was too much fuel to put them out with plain old water; we'd need foam to smother the fire's base, but it was good enough for now.

The foreman pointed at his watch, flashed two gloved fingers and then pointed up. He added a garbled "Inutes."

I gathered it would take two more minutes to get to the top, so I told Command to reduce the pressure again so we could move the hose with us and that the next task force would need some foam. I also told them I was sending two of my men back who were low on air. Everybody else including myself had enough for another 10 to 15 minutes. We were about 55 feet up.

Once we were ready, we began to shuffle back up the catwalk, one hand on everyone's back, the foreman leading the way. Eight were now six and the six were scared shitless.

Excerpt from Incident Commander's Summary

The building was divided up into three groups with three task forces created to hunt and extinguish the fires. Task Force 1 was sent with a Solid Waste Manager since the workers were certain there were fires in the main trash area and at the top of the complex. TF1 extinguished the fire in the main area and then moved to the top informing Command a overhaul crew would need foam to put out all the spot fires completely. Little fire was noted at the top and TF1 left the hose and moved to Rehab to rest (see Lt. Braunworth's injury report).

I guessed we had to be pretty close to the top when our caravan seemed to bog down. We were back in darkness, although I could see something hanging down in front of us; it was heavy, thick and black. Without much discussion we followed the lead, pushing past this weight with our heads and shoulders bearing the burden. Finally it blocked us completely.

"—veyer belt," the foreman yelled back. "We...cut it–"

A tap came on my shoulder. "—ose is suck-"

My air mask vocabulary took it in. From what I gathered one of the conveyer belts was in our way and we were out of hose. It always has amazed how 200 feet of hose can be used up with 10 feet here, a corner here and there and then after 60 feet of elevation suddenly you needed more. It never seemed to add up.

I okayed the cutting of the conveyer belt and called Command to stop the pump so we could add 50 feet of rolled hose one of the new guys was given to carry. I hoped it would be enough to get us where we were going. Once again to do this I had to open the side of me mask in order to speak clearly into the mic of the radio.

We checked airpacks. We all had about ten minutes except for one of the new guys. He was down to 600 psi. I sent him and the other new guy back as a precaution and told Command. Duncan sawed away at the conveyer belt with a large pocket knife. As the final strands were hacked at, it slumped some more, sagged onto all of us, and finally dropped 65 feet to the floor of the building. When this happened we clung to each other so that if it took one of us down it would take everybody. We were left with sore necks and still a pile of conveyer belt impeding our way.

To continue, we couldn't walk on the catwalk since there was about eight rubbery folds still lying there, so we went hand over hand on the guardrail with feet dangling over a smoky floor and a limp hose squeezed under our necks, until we could pull ourselves back up onto a stairwell for the last rung of the journey.

What we found was a 10 by 10 foot work area with a smoldering fire waiting to die having exhausted all its fuel. "This is it?" I wanted to ask, but never got it out. I felt something in my back, something familiar I should know.

My Air pack had only 500 psi of air left, and hopefully, just enough to get out. Everyone else's air was at least 800 so I told the men to put this fire out and get back to the ground ASAP. Tipping my air mask once more, I told Command to increase the pump pressure just before I gave Duncan the radio and bid farewell.

Tired and agitated, I began to make the long trek back to firm ground and fresh air. Hand over hand past the "veyer belt" and then I searched for the handrail through the darkness. I hustled, making the most of my time, sensing it was getting harder to breathe, the air pack telling me through my lungs it was getting lower and lower. I was into the main trash room with not much further to go. My lungs were now heavy and I picked up the pace.

Although I noticed some spot fires still flaring up on occasion, I tried to keep my eyes on the catwalk. My airpack was now wheezing; my head ached and my lungs were not getting enough air. I was coming up to more darkness and as I recalled, no handrails.

There was no way other than crawling to assure I didn't fall, so on all fours I scurried like a mouse feeling the hard, warmed metal through my bunker pants and gloves. I stopped when my air mask was sucked against my face.

It's funny the things you remember in a crisis situation. Things you hadn't thought about in years, or ever really thought about. I remember in the fire academy we had practiced "buddy breathing". Undoing our hoses to our masks and hooking up to a "buddy's" mask or bottle in smoke-filled darkness.

I remembered one of students asking the instructor what to do if you were all by yourself.

Quickly, I undid my hose and tucked it into the armpit of my coat. The smoke I did take in was thick and pasty, tasting of rubber and metal, making me gag. I continued on, realizing I had to get out in the next few minutes or my memorial would be the subject of some firefighter video about do's and don'ts.

I continued to crawl, now hugging the metal harder, knowing I would soon become disoriented due to lack of oxygen. I couldn't see at all since the heat from my body was now fogging my mask. Every once in a while I'd accidentally pinch my hose with my arm or chest and my mask would get sucked against my face, then I'd have to stop and readjust, getting a whiff of smoke on occasion which irritated my lungs so much I would hack uncontrollably. My head was pounding now and I felt as if I couldn't continue, but I knew I had to. I'd seen too many videos and read too many

gg5555599999999999999bbb

articles in which firefighters had suffocated three feet from the right way out or been so lost they didn't know they were within reach of an stairwell. I couldn't be more than 30 feet from ground level. Thirty feet! What else could I do, anyway? Maybe catch the new guys I'd just released? No, they were too far ahead. Wait for Duncan and the rest? No- if I did that, I'd definitely be in one of those videos.

I crawled as fast as I could, now coughing on a regular basis. At one point I thought maybe I could go faster with my hose dragging along outside, but the lack of clean air paralyzed me. There had to be handrails and light soon.

I knew I wasn't going fast anymore. Slow motion was the best I could do.

Boom, boom, boom. My head pounded away. All my muscles ached and I was so tired. Maybe just a little rest. Maybe just lay here on the warmed catwalk for a minute. No! God, let me keep going. I reached with my hands and pulled my body along the metal with all the strength I could muster. Boom, boom, boom. Just a little rest. Oh, God help me. And then something stopped me. Boom, boom, boom. I felt it; it was rubber, it was sticky, it went up. It was a—

"Ay, wha the–" I heard somebody mutter through an air mask.

I was pulled up with gloved hands. My mask was fogged; I was seeing little sparklies every once in a while. "Bren— wha da—"

I was asleep and this had to be a dream. I was taking my last breaths and this is what my mind wanted to believe. This was the fire's final illusion.

"Mon, mon," said the mirage.

I went through the motions to make friends with the mirage. *Okay here's my hose I'll put it in your mask. I need air. Happy?*

"Mon, mon. Rab da rail..."

Okay, okay- I'll play along. Let's go. Not too fast. Oh, that was where the rail was!

Then it hit me I was moving. Fresh, bottled air had cleared my mask. I took a closer look at the mirage. "Tony," I said. "Tony Johnson."

"Mon, le's go—"

That slight bit of air had cleared my head a little, although I could tell it still wasn't enough though for my body. I began to be the impetus to move faster. We turned a corner. There, I saw light: it was either Heaven or the outside. I ripped my hose away from Tony and went sprinting down the catwalk, eventually diving out onto the ground and into dusk's finale for the day.

My mask came off first, then my coat. I was soaked with sweat and coughing up black rubbery, metallic-tasting foam and sputum. Somebody grabbed me and ran me over to a rescue truck. Oxygen was jammed in my face.

I looked up and saw Tony Johnson, one of the guys I'd sent back who'd been low on air. "I changed my air bottle and was just coming back to see if you guys needed any more help. I thought I heard something so I started banging on the handrail with my light," he said.

It's funny how the mind rationalizes everything. I would have made it even without help, I told myself, sitting in a rehab area drinking water. Nah, I didn't need to go to the hospital- it wasn't that bad. Sure, I know I shouldn't have been traveling by myself, but hell- it was only a garbage fire. No big deal.

The next day at about 6:00 p.m., I started burning up. In the hospital that night I found out I had pneumonia. I was out for five weeks.

Excerpts from Memo By Lt. Brent Braunworth

....and furthermore there was no reason to ever go into that type of environment at that point. It was wrong of Command to send us in without floor plans and no idea of what we were getting into. There was literally no briefing and no appropriate back up.....

Years later I can sit back and laugh at it and admit that if Tony hadn't come along I would have died. I can chuckle and tell lies with friends about the Great Garbage Scow Fire and what a great hero I was. Hell, it took the crews all night to put out all the little fires in that place.

However, I'll never forget the creepy feeling of trying but not caring of whether I died or not. The feeling of giving up scares me to this day; how so quickly a strong, invincible young man can be reduced to a babbling mess.

And sometimes when I'm dozing in a lounger reading Travis Magee in the wee hours of the morning after a call, I get that feeling....Through the heat and smoke I can't breathe, my muscles are aching. I can't make it. Boom, boom, boom. I'm crawling, sleepy.

Boom, boom, boom.

Suddenly I am awake. "God? Tony?"

Not just the TV and the Three Stooges.

Child's Play

Looking back, it seems like we were on "hydrant test."

To make sure water pressure is high enough to fight a fire, one has to wrench loose a huge, often extremely tight bolt to free a stream of water from the hydrant. The work is sweaty and monotonous and for some reason done in the hottest of months. And, of course, there are hundreds in our city. Consequently, my partner and I were more than happy to abandon the routine to respond to a "drowning" in the south end of town.

Back then I had only about a year's experience with the fire department and two years as a paramedic, so it was all kind of new and exciting.

But this call would begin a metamorphosis, and what was new, fun and exciting would soon become just a job.

We stopped at an older, little house east of Dixie Highway, not far from where West Palm Beach ends and Lake Worth begins. As I hurried to get the equipment we'd need, I noticed the house was kind of homey with a potpourri of child's toys decorating the front yard.

As we entered the front door, the tension settled on us like a heavy backpack. A little boy was lying limp and lifeless on the patio next to a covered pool. Our guys hovered over him, reciting standing orders and frantically searching for equipment while performing CPR. There were other people inside the house whom I took to be family and concerned neighbors, yelling and crying, and one gray-haired old lady who kept saying, "I only took my eyes off of him for a minute. I don't know how-"

The little boy was no more than three, with blond hair and blue eyes - a beautiful little boy. His skin was pale, his Winnie the Pooh matching shirt and shorts outfit was soaked and dripping. His tiny hands were in the same clutching position they must have been in as he tried and tried to hold on to the side of the above-ground pool.

I was sorry for everyone in the room, including us.

The lead medic of the other crew shouted over to us, "He's almost three. Somehow he got into the covered pool. The parents have been called." The medic paused from his compressions to check for a pulse. He shook his head and started again. "Our truck broke down. We need yours."

It looked like the other crew had already established an IV in the boy's arm and CPR was being done adequately, so I went to the airway. There was a probationary medic at the head. "We can't intubate him," he said. "Everybody's tried."

What he was talking about was placing a tube down the boy's trachea to better ventilate the lungs. It's kind of tricky in kids, but essential. I didn't have a lot of experience with pediatrics, but I knew that this was the key to this type of call. If I could intubate this boy, he might have a chance.

I took over the ventilations and bided my time until I could get a chance to perform the procedure. We quickly transferred the boy to our stretcher and after we got him to the back of our truck, our driver took off like a bat out of hell for the hospital.

The other lead medic was still doing compressions, having decided to ride with us to Good Samaritan Hospital. He had opted to go instead of my older partner. Since my partner had been on so many of these types of calls, he was more than happy to avoid all of the trauma and turmoil you had when a child died. That was one thing I'd noticed: the older you got, the more hardened you became on most calls, except for those with kids. I've seen medics nearly quit their jobs after serious calls involving children. It was almost too stressful, too close to the edge.

I prepared to take a look in the boy's mouth with a

laryngoscope, a tool that not only moves the tongue out of the way but allows the medic to see the beginning of the trachea because of a bright light located light on the end of it. Most kids' tracheae are much higher up compared to those in adults. It's considered extremely difficult, so I prepared myself.

I was nervous, my hands shaking slightly. I stopped ventilating the boy and began the procedure.

"What're you doin'?" said the other medic. His eyes were moist; he had three kids of his own.

"I think I can tube him," I said, straining to lift up on the boy's mouth with the tool. I thought I could see it but with every bump in the road the elusive trachea disappeared. I got the tube ready. I waited patiently and once it appeared again I jammed the plastic device into place.

"You're wastin' your time—"

I cut him off. "I think I got it."

I continued to ventilate as he listened to the boy's lungs with the stethoscope eventually saying, "You're in. Good job, kid."

I felt good and extremely lucky. I knew this little boy had a chance now. I pumped in syringes of epinephrine one after another using the IV and the tube as we rocked and rolled in the back of the rescue truck. The other medic was dripping with sweat as he made every compression count.

He stopped and checked a pulse while I continued to breathe for the boy. "I got complexes on the ECG," he said. "I think I got a pulse." I saw normal beats run across the face of the ECG monitor.

His eyes were still moist, but he smiled. He raised his hand and I gave him a high five. I smiled, too. I knew we wouldn't let the family down.

I recalled the only other time I'd saved a child. It was another three-year-old, but one who had Down's Syndrome and a whole bunch of other medical problems. I ended up getting a pulse back on him, too, but unfortunately that only meant he would die two weeks later in the hospital after eating up all of his parent's life savings. I remembered his parents. They took it all nonchalantly, just kind of nodding when I told them their son would be okay. They had seen that before; they had been through everything before.

I must have seemed young and foolish.

But this kid really would be okay, I thought. *He would make it and I actually made a difference.*

The other medic kept feeling the pulse. "I'm losing it," he said. I watched as the beats on the ECG monitor became fewer and fewer. He felt the neck again. "What's going on? No pulse!" he screamed.

Start CPR," I said. "Check the lungs." We were just pulling into the hospital.

"Let's go! Let's go!" somebody was yelling.

We hustled the stretcher into the main room in the back of the ER doing CPR as best as we could while we ran. We lifted him onto the hospital stretcher and let the pediatric experts take over.

I was sweating and breathing heavy as I watched them work. The other medic went outside to put the truck back in order. He hadn't looked at me when he walked out; I guess he foresaw the inevitable.

I still had hope.

They pushed drug after drug, but no pulse returned. In between CPR they turned the boy and prodded him all over to see if there was some other underlying problem.

Finally, they stopped. "It's no use," said one of the doctors. "He's been down too long."

I felt empty, drained and cheated. I wanted him to live; I needed some sense of right or good to come out of this. He had his whole life ahead of him. Why a boy? Why couldn't it have been just another cardiac arrest from a nursing home? Why?

I remember walking outside. It was all kind of dreamlike. The family was all there, even the parents. All eyes were on me, searching for some kind of sign, I'm sure, although I'm certain that with all the medics coming in and out of the ER, they didn't know I was the one who had been with their boy.

You could tell they were sensing their worst nightmare had come true.

Grandma was sitting on a bench, her head in her hands, tears pouring down her fingers like raindrops. It wasn't hard to pick out the mother: she was the young, hysterical woman who, like me, kept asking "Why?"

I avoided their stares until I met the father's gaze. His eyes were sad, but he wasn't crying. He stood there, hands in his pockets, looking obliviously at everything that passed by him.

When our eyes met, I could see his pain and sadness. It was a vacuous look, like he didn't know what to do or what was really going on and one that made me think that if he lost his son, he might never do anything constructive again– like an old fighter who survived a horrendous beating but still had to wait for a decision.

A father should never be asked to bury his son.

I knew how he felt, in a way, because I was a man, too, but I could never relate to his pain. For a moment he appeared as if he was going to ask me a question and I quickly looked away and walked off. It was a time for religion and silence.

And I would never forget it.

Eight years later and I still toss and turn in a deep sleep yelling out, "I think I got it!" and "Check the lungs!"

Like a nightmare, I remember everything perfectly and relive it. Rolling around in the back of the truck. A little, motionless body on a stretcher. A father's eyes.

I have a son now and I try to spend as much time with him as possible. At times I think it's just an attempt to create "moments" because paramedics are reminded everyday that life can dangle by a single thread, that a life can become a memory in a matter of seconds and the only thing you have left afterwards are those "moments."

Sometimes at night, I find myself waking up and going to his room while he's sleeping and I hug him so tightly he wakes up.

He has blond hair, too.

More times than not, when I'm holding him, I start to cry and I hear my three year old son say, "Dad, what's wrong?" like an adult.

And I can't stop crying and I can't reply and he holds my head, saying, "Dad, it'll be okay. It's not that bad."

Occasionally while I lie there, I feel myself going through yet another metamorphosis. I am reduced to a child in a man's body, scared of covered pools and people in uniforms, and I hug my son that much tighter.

A Duty To Act

It was not a new story by any means. A man and a woman together for almost half a century and then, in their twilight years when life should be its simplest, the worst happens: one gets cancer- not a cancer that takes her life immediately, but a cancer that lingers, causing more and more pains as it grows.

So, together they plotted and planned their own suicide. Not a violent one, but an overdose, one to ease the pain of both of them, to stop the cancer and let them be together, because he could not bear to live without her.

It was about 9:00 a.m. and we were at the station having just finished checking out the Rescue truck, when we got the call. It came in as a double suicide—a possible overdose—but we responded only one paramedic unit anyway—my unit.

When I got there, I found an elderly gentleman slumped in a chair holding hands with a woman who lay on her back in a hospital bed. Both were still warm and both were pulseless. I immediately called for another unit and began to work the two patients with my partners.

I had no history or knowledge of the cancer until right before the second truck arrived. A neighbor came in, rattling out their story. The wife had had cancer for two years and her husband could not bear to see her in such pain or be without her. "Their love," she said, "was that strong." She was the one who called 911.

I paused for a moment thinking, like a man not a medic. I thought about things like a fifty year love, slow death by cancer, and two people who had made a mature, mutual decision. Lastly, I thought about leaving them alone.

Would it be so wrong? If we were thinking either legally or ethically, yes, but what about morally? These two people had been together longer than I had been on this earth and with all the years of their experience they had chosen this decision. Why couldn't I let them carry it out?

It was society that had made the rule that no one shall take their own life or another's, but could society have possibly examined all the different factors that come into play in a case like this? This was obviously not a spur of the moment decision; it had been well thought out. The pill bottles were just not tossed aside but sitting on the bedside table. Their house was well-kept. The husband had dressed his wife in a new bed gown and he was in a nice shirt and slacks. This was how they wanted to go, to be remembered. Legally, suicide is wrong; ethically, I should continue to work on them. Morally, I was torn.

I wondered if I could ever love someone that much.

But the duty to act kicked in, the legal doctrine that requires paramedics help the sick and injured to the best of their ability in any situation. More legal terms flooded my mind, things like implied consent and negligence. How could I let them die? I wasn't programmed that way; it was against everything I'd been taught.

All eyes were on me as I made my decision, an unforgivable decision in some eyes. I shrugged off my feelings and began to bark out orders.

The other medics arrived and I directed them to the husband since I was already with the wife. We had CPR going on both on them and equipment seemed to be flying everywhere.

I placed a tube down her trachea and started an IV in her arm. I administered drug after drug, strictly by the book, until I noticed a shockable rhythm on the heart monitor.

Picking up the paddles, I was again overwhelmed by those feelings. In a job that should personify the epitome of compassion I've learned that sometimes you have to turn everything off and become almost robotic.

Taking a deep breath, I got back to work. I shocked her twice with the paddles and her body twisted and convulsed in response to the electricity. Finally, I heard the words that I most didn't want to hear.

"Hey- I feel a pulse," said one of my partners.

We took her to the hospital; the other squad took him.

During the ride the wife even began to breathe again on her own, four or five times a minute. Another definite sign of recovery, but for some reason, I wasn't very happy about it.

She ended up surviving, but her husband was pronounced a few minutes after the doctor saw him.

It was a nightmare come true. I couldn't sleep that night. More disturbing questions were on my mind. Does a paramedic's duty to act supersede all moral and personal obligations? Should I have just left them alone? What gave me the right to alter their lives, or in this case, their deaths?

Fifty years of love, and then love enough to die together. I again wondered if I could ever love someone that much.

I came to only one conclusion that sleepless night: that sometimes this job could be the worst.

The next morning I went home, trying to forget the call. I found some solace in bourbon but more in thought. Who or what gave me the right to play God? My decision was unforgivable and maybe damnable, but if you damned me you'd have to damn the entire system, both medical and legal.

I thought a lot about the husband and wife. As a paramedic you tend to treat the elderly in certain situations kind of like children, as if they were unaware of what was going on. You don't condescend to them, but rather you talk above them. Instead of letting them make a decision solely on their own, you direct them, thinking that because of your youth you know best. After this call I knew I would never take the elderly for granted again. It was obvious to me that their emotions were just as deep-seated and focused as my own. They, with their experience and knowledge, were probably more aware of what was important in life than even I was.

I drank a lot and early that morning so I could sleep and not dream. I was worried, worried I'd dream about a woman I'd saved, saved so she could spend the rest of her life in a mental institution contemplating the futility of her own existence, as she longed for her spouse and cringed in pain every few minutes, because of her loss and because of the painful disease inside her.

Crimson Eyes

I was there to help him, if he needed it. He lay on his side with his face turned toward the clouds, eyes wide, red and non-blinking. Singed hair and eyebrows hung over those eyes. A light smoke and the pungent smell of gasoline, the two things that eventually did him in, still hung in the air.

As I looked around the room you could see that he tried to claw his way out through the drywall when he was unable to find a door. What a way to go.

"Can ya do anything?"

I looked down and his crimson eyes seemed to burn mine like lasers.

"Can ya do anything?" the Captain repeated.

"No," I said. "He's gone."

"Shame," said another voice. "He coulda been a helluva fireman."

It had been a solid day at #3 Fire station, complete with a number of assaults, a chest pain and even a stabbing, boy versus boy. By the time dinner came around we were buried in paperwork and starving. My partner, Mike Curry, was handling most of it while I prepared the food we had picked up earlier at the store.

"One down," he hollered as he forged away at the mountain of legal documentation that was an obvious necessity to everyone but the boys who did it.

"Keep up the good work," I yelled back. I was outside

just getting ready to put the chicken quarters on the grill. *It takes time,* I rationalized, feeling guilty I didn't have a report in hand, *to prepare chicken just right.*

The Captain, Kenny, the youngest one at the time to ever make it, ventured outside making small talk. "Did you put that chicken on yet?"

"No, why? You hungry?"

He paused, sniffing the wind. "No. I smell something burning..."

I turned my nose into the wind. "Great," I said, hauling the food inside. "Hold on; I'll go with ya."

So with me in charge of rescue and young Captain Kenny following his nose on the pumper we set off together idling slowly forward with our trucks, cruising the streets of West Palm in search of the ultimate goal of a firefighter: the working structure fire.

"What the hell are we doin'?" Curry howled from the back of the rescue truck, no doubt angry from being interrupted from his paperwork and his subsequent dinner.

"Mike, my first partner told me once to never doubt the nose of a real fireman when it comes to either fires or food."

"Did you smell it?"

"No."

At that moment the tones went off. "Engine 3, Rescue 3, respond to a structure fire in the area of 700 39th Street."

We followed the pumper, screaming down a back alley until we got to within two blocks of the address, then I told my driver to pick it up around the corner. The smell was now strong and I could see what appeared to be smoke in the night sky.

"Curry, we got one," I said.

"I'm almost ready." I could hear him rolling around back there frantically trying to get on his bunker gear and air pack. At this point, he could well have stopped since my driver and I still needed to dress fully and it was against SOP to report for assignment to a fire scene Commander without your whole unit. The more people who were with you at a fire, the safer you were when a problem occurred.

I guided my driver down a side street so the engine could lay a supply line from the hydrant without us getting in the way.

Flames were shooting out the back of a one-story wooden house. The dark smoke which makes fire investigators cringe was billowing from the fire, rising high and disappearing into the cloudless night sky.

I slid into my bunker gear—boots, pants, coat and helmet—and slung an air pack over my shoulder. After making sure my crew was dressed to the hilt, we hustled over to Kenny who was already on the radio for more units.

The fire was so staggering he was on a leader line himself protecting an exposure, in this case the closest house next door, so it wouldn't catch fire as well. He directed my driver to take over for him and told me and Mike to grab the other leader line and move around back, putting out what we could of the actual fire itself.

The smell of gasoline was biting as we moved into the backyard. It was pitch black and, with radio in hand, I kept tripping over the inch and three-quarter attack hose as we stretched it out. At less than 2 inches in diameter this type of hose was easy to maneuver, either wet or dry. As I did this, I could hear other units responding to the fire on the radio.

"Give us water! Give us water!" Curry was yelling. Embers were falling, stinging the backs of our necks.

"Let's hook up," I said. Like two singled-minded drones, we dropped the limp hose in order to place our air masks on and hooked up our bottled air. Our actions were simultaneous due to good training. We picked up the hose again and waited. More and more smoke drifted in our direction; pieces of flaming wood tumbled down from the sky.

Finally, we could feel the hose get hard in our hands. With no prompting, Mike took the lead and I fed him the line as he commenced fighting the fire.

As many fires as I have gone to, I am still amazed how

much a little water can do.

Even when things are apparently insurmountable and it seems the whole world is ablaze, once the water gets flowing things get dramatically better.

I guess that's common sense, but from where I stood that night, we put out 30 foot flames shooting out the back of the house in a matter of seconds.

Soon the flames were gone and there was just a humid, smoky, sodden feel to the back of the house. We tried to open a back door but it was locked up tight. From what he could see inside through a window with cupped hands, Curry said he thought there was a 2x4 across the inside of it. I just shrugged since our bells were going off, signifying that our air bottles were too low to continue and for right now the fire was over for us, so we handed the hose over to the grumbling fire-medics of Rescue 1 as they came around the corner and we left for a much deserved break.

I was exhausted. We'd been pretty steady that day, all very typical for the north end of West Palm. I'd also gotten in an intense workout in the weight room after lunch. Consequently, I wasn't enthused when Kenny told me on the radio to ventilate the back room.

Curry and I hustled since the idea of a backdraft—an explosion in a confined area due to the entrance of air to an oxygen starved environment—is terrifying and dangerous for firefighters and we didn't want that guilt on our shoulders, but we were bitching something awful when we laddered the building after noting there had to be ten fresh guys sitting out in staging, drinking water. I figured it was all in a day's work and kept pacifying myself by thinking I'd be off in less than twelve hours.

Once on the roof I took the first ten whacks with the axe, making just a little hole the size of my fist in the roof.

"Gimme that!" Curry bellowed. "You work out so much, you're weak when I need ya."

As much as he complained you could see the pleasure in

his eyes whenever he was working hard. Me, I'd been to too many fires and it was just dirty, unglamorous work.

Curry had soon etched out a hole double the size of the one I'd put in. Hot, toxic air spewed forth, releasing the built up gases which might cause an explosion. Curry was going to do more, but I'd heard too many war stories from the old ones, about firefighters falling into flames from charred, sagging roofs to allow it. This would be good enough.

Back out front, I managed to get a glass of water from one of the guys standing around watching. From where I was standing it seemed like guys were just starting to enter the building. I approached Kenny, saying, "What gives? Haven't you guys searched yet?"

Normally, we would have been searching for fire victims as the fire was being extinguished.

"It was all boarded up," he said, radio close to his ear. "All except for one door. I gotta crew inside now for about two minutes."

We both heard it on the radio together. "I—we—got somebody down—I dunno—I need medics—"

Curry was already on it when he saw me move to the house and I waved him over to the door, listening to him say, "Why not? We've already done everything else."

I quickly explained the situation as we headed inside the house, suggesting it was probably a little firefighter heat exhaustion; it happens all the time. Sometimes the heavy clothes we use to protect us can also work against us. Too much heat under that kind of insulation and your body's thermometer goes haywire.

It was thick with wet heat, but the smoke was nearly all gone so there was no need to hook up our air masks. Firefighters with sad eyes met us and waved us to a back room.

The Captain approached me as I entered. The walls had been charred, but there had been no fire here. With no explanation he pointed to the middle of the floor. There in a heap of human jelly lay a man.

"What do ya think?" asked the Captain removing his own air mask.

I was there to help him, if he needed it. He lay on his side with his face turned toward the clouds, eyes wide, red and non-blinking. A light smoke and the pungent smell of gasoline, the two things that did him in, still hung in the air.

As I looked around the room you could see where he tried to claw his way out through drywall when he was unable to find a door. What a way to go.

"Can ya do anything?"

I looked down and his crimson eyes seemed to burn mine like lasers.

"Can ya do anything?" the Captain repeated.

"No," I said. "He's gone."

"Shame," said another voice. "He coulda been a helluva fireman."

There were hardened chuckles in the background.

He was a light Hispanic male about forty wearing blue jeans and a tee shirt.

It's hard enough to catch arsonists, let alone to catch the one who hired him. I had learned that in an arson investigation class I took. Arsonists are usually hired hands who, immediately after the act, drift into the background while the owner sits with friends or business associates up to his eyebrows with a good alibi.

The insurance company fights it, but without proof they usually always pay, and the owner walks away with big bucks, leaving an unrentable home for the city to clean up.

"I think we found your arsonist," I said.

No fire death is ever good, even if it is the bad guy. Usually, they are charred pieces of meat left on the grill too long. Their skin slides off their arms when you try to move them; they are hairless and bubbled. One never forgets the smell of burnt flesh; it is the smell of death. There's even a taste to it, a taste that lingers in the mouth for days.

Initially though, before the fire takes over cooking your

body, you die like this guy did- mind panicking, lungs burning, eyes and nose watering until finally you take a breath and there's no air in it at all and your chest feels like it's ready to explode and then you give up knowingly. You lie down content with the feeling that you will soon see blackness and sleep forever. I've been close to that, so I know.

"How do ya know for sure?"

"Well, for one thing," I began, turning away from the laser eyes. "He's still clutching what he used to light it off in his hands." I pointed to his left one, fingers were still wrapped around a pack of matches. "It looks like after he got done spreading the gasoline around, he lit the back room first and then went to light this one up before leaving, but it was too thick with fumes in here so when he lit the match the room flashed over instead of catching fire. It blinded him and when he couldn't find the door handle he panicked and tried to claw his way out, then he just suffocated. Better call an investigator."

"Thanks, doc," said the Captain.

Curry and I walked outside, leaving the rest of them inside.

Only about seven per cent of my job is actual firefighting, the medic calls are a lot more frequent. I've had some close calls working as a paramedic, but there is nothing more crazy and dangerous than running into a burning building when everybody's natural instinct is to run out. Firefighters die each year, just like that arsonist, terrible air-hungry, suffocating, lonely deaths. Then the fire takes over, charring, baking and twisting your body.

I've attended a few funerals.

"Let's get outa here," I said, shaking my head. "Poor bastard."

"A lot of people might say he got what he deserved," Curry replied.

"Nobody deserves to die like that," I mused. "I hope he got paid first and had some fun."

We moved to the truck. Our driver was already there, his

bunker gear by his side.

"Ready to go back and cook that chicken?" he asked.

I swung my airpack from my back to the ground. "No, I think I'll pass. I'm not real hungry anymore."

Touch Of The Master's Hand

The call came in as a "Fall- woman needs help back into bed", addressed at a semi-ritzy house near the water. As my partner and I got into the ambulance we were praying there would be no injuries and thus be canceled for two reasons: fatigue—we worked the night before, and the AC in our truck was on the fritz and this being South Florida in the summer we thought if we kept running calls we might be the next patients lugged into the ER with heat stroke.

As my partner slowly headed toward the beach, I made the futile effort of hammering on the dash with the hope of some reciprocal cool air, but instead it just seemed to get hotter.

"Damn! I just don't seem to have the magic touch," I whined, knowing full well the "old man", also known as the owner of the company, would have to hit it just once to get compliance from the compressor.

Sweating, we waited as patiently as we could for the Boynton Beach Fire Rescue unit to cancel us. No such luck- we knew Boynton was breaking in a new medic, so we weren't surprised things were moving a little slower than usual.

It was a modest little mansion catty-cornered to a playground. When we arrived, the patient was still sitting on the floor talking to Tommy, the new medic. She had a contusion on her forehead but was refusing to go to the hospital. The lady's private nurse, a Filipino, was hovering close by with a wary eye on these four strange men, every once in a while blurting out items of the patient's medical history.

The old lady looked to be about two-hundred-years-old and obviously realized any ride to the hospital could be her last. Tommy was asking all the right questions and she was giving all the right answers:

"Did you lose consciousness?"

"No."

"Do you have any neck or back pain?"

"No."

"Do you want to go to the hospital?"

"No."

This didn't leave the new medic much choice, knowing full well that he was being scrutinized by everyone and that the old lady should probably go and get checked out.

"Well," he began cautiously. "I guess if you don't wanna go you don't have to," he sighed, playing the part of a caring medic who really needed this job. "But let's just see how you feel standing up."

Slowly, he stood her up. "How do ya feel?"

She nodded as if she was okay, but didn't seem exactly rock steady.

"Let's see how ya do walking." She looked like an intoxicated Frankenstein monster as she made her way across the floor.

Tommy wasn't exactly happy with her uncoordinated, robotic movements.

"Ma'am," he said. "Maybe we oughta take ya up- you don't seem real steady."

About this time the nurse came back into the room and had what can best be described as (so far as advanced medical terminology goes) a conniption. She began to holler in Filipino and seemingly froth at the mouth. I thought we had another medical alarm.

"Oh my God," the nurse, fanning herself, finally exclaimed in English. "She's had polio all her life and those are the first steps she's taken in thirty years!!!"

You could see all the blood rush from Tommy's face. All he could manage was, "oh, uh, in that case then, I guess she can stay."

We waited by our ambulance for the Boynton squad to come outside. My partner and I had requests. He had a trick knee and a headache that needed healing and I was hoping Tommy could just lay his hand on the engine and fix the AC.

But as usual we were out of luck. Smiling, he waved us off, explaining he couldn't possibly waste the powers of his hands on mere ambulance jockeys.

Real Men

It can catch you anywhere, the thousand yard stare. You become so engrossed in thought you stop what you're doing and literally lose track of time. From what I've seen most paramedics do it. You relive certain calls: what you did right, what you did wrong, how you felt.

I'm no different: this time it catches me about 1 a.m., right after I shower as I'm toweling off.....

The call came in as a rollover on I-95, northbound lane in the north end of the city. That day I was "stepped up" to EMS Captain- better known as the shift supervisor- of all the paramedics riding on the rescue trucks.

A day in that position usually starts off kind of slow with a lot of administrative work but normally builds. It was around noon and having done the "paperwork shuffle" for the last three hours, I was happy for the break to run a call.

Rescue 5, Engine 5 and EMS 2 (my unit) were dispatched. One good thing about this position was that you got to avoid the ridiculous complaints such as foot pains, headaches, and arthritis for three days. As EMS Captain you only went to serious calls.

Over the years I've noticed only about one out of every ten calls like this are actually rollovers and an even less of a percentage of that have injuries. Most of the time even if it is a rollover the occupants are already milling around the scene by the time we get there, more worried about the damage to their cars than their health.

As soon as I got in my truck I robotically called dispatch to see if Riviera Beach Fire, the department to the north, was going. I knew they probably were, since it was part of an automatic aid agreement in an attempt to give quicker emergency medical care to accident victims, but I asked anyway.

Surprisingly, I was told that they were not responding and that it was definitely our call. No problem, I figured, one out of ten.

I was about three miles out when Rescue 5 arrived. About 30 seconds later a harried voice called me on the radio. "Rescue 5, EMS 2: we have a rollover with three or four serious injuries. We'll prep the worst one for transport." It was a bad sign; my guys never get excited.

I began to bark out some orders, or better yet reminders. It was my job to coordinate the scene and suggest patient care, not necessarily to perform it. Rescue 5 didn't reply as they had their hands full.

Engine 5 arrived and the Captain took Command of the scene, stating they were assisting in the assessment of the other patients.

Traffic was now picking up on 95 and I was almost to the end of our city limits. The rubberneckers were in full force making me swerve, use the emergency lane and almost causing me to get in an accident myself.

When I was out of the city I called back to dispatch and told them to send Riviera, explaining that although it was close it wasn't our call. I was now antsy wanting to get there, find out it really wasn't that bad and turf the paperwork to Riviera when they arrived.

I know it's selfish, but paramedics are so overburdened with reports and addendums and releases that this is how we think.

I arrived at the scene throwing my car in park, placing it in the emergency lane going northbound directly parallel with Engine 5 who was in one of the three southbound lanes blocking traffic. As I hopped across the median I could only see blue shirts and yellow bunker pants huddled in several different areas: no car or no victims yet.

As I got closer I saw some of my guys coming toward me, rolling a stretcher. It was the driver and Lieutenant of Rescue 5 moving very quickly. I made eye contact with the lieutenant and he gave me the scoop on the run. "There are three serious traumas," he said. He dipped his head toward the bloodied body on the stretcher. "This one went through the front side passenger window. He's the worst, but the others are pretty bad, too. I left my second medic Kevin with one of them. I didn't let St. Mary's know yet."

I looked down at a non-moving body dressed in a bathing suit and a T-shirt with only one shoe. He was young but you couldn't tell his age; almost his entire head had been bandaged and blood was soaking through. I rubbed his sternum to get a response; there was none.

It was an obvious head injury. "Let's get him tubed and hyperventilate him. Why don't you try to do it en route?" He nodded knowingly, moving on to his truck which was parked about 100 feet behind mine.

I turned back and broke into a run. Now I could take in the entire scene: the car was upright in the middle lane. Some of the front roof looked to have been torn while the back part was crushed. The windshield was shattered and missing large chunks like something had exploded through it.

The Captain of Engine 5 approached me as I neared. His people were assessing two other victims. I told him I would assume Command and to have the Highway Patrol block all southbound and northbound traffic since we might need the helicopter. He explained it was one of the worst accidents he'd ever seen and that they were all kids. I could see the pain in his eyes. I knew him and there was no real reason for myself to question this; he had seen his fair share of death so as I moved onward I jumped on the radio.

I let the local trauma center, St. Mary's Hospital, know Rescue 5 was en route with an young adult male who was unconscious and asked if they could take two more traumas. They said they could only take one. I told dispatch to respond two more rescue trucks and then called for the County transport chopper, A.K.A. the Traumahawk. One of these kids had to go Delray Community 25 miles south.

There were firefighters and fire-medics in two different areas. As I walked to the scene I gathered that whomever had been driving had swerved to miss some debris in the middle lane. It looked like a plastic pot you might put medium-sized plants in. It then appeared the car had lost control, flipped and eventually rolled over several times.

I finally reached the first patient, a young male, probably eighteen. He was semi-conscious, lying on his side, babbling the same questions over and over: "Who are you guys? Who are you guys? Where's the car? Where's the car?"

The engine guys were dressing his head with some thick gauze since he was bleeding steadily from some laceration buried deep in his hair. His left leg was possibly broken and every few moments he would spasmodically cough up a trickle of blood which he wiped on his sleeve.

"Who are you guys? Who are you guys?"

"He said he crawled from the car," somebody said. "Kevin's with the girl, she's worse."

I quickly helped them get the boy on a backboard and called to see how far out my other rescues were. When I left they were placing him on oxygen and attempting to splint his leg.

A truck of Riviera Fire-medics pulled up and they scrambled over to me and the boy. They could take him to St. Mary's immediately. As they took over care one of them said another rescue was on the way.

I grabbed a firefighter and we hustled over to the girl. It was only about twenty feet, but it seemed like it took me forever to get there. It appeared that here, on this scene, where time was of utmost importance, I could do nothing fast.

When we got there what I saw made me take a few steps back. She was a beautiful girl, an eighteen-year-old Barbie Doll who looked like she'd been cut head to toe with a razor blade. She was covered in blood, most of it coming from an open head wound on the left side of her head. I now knew *who* had been driving and *what* had exploded through the front windshield.

Kevin was holding her head trying to place a c-collar on her neck by himself. My first thought was *she's got to be dead*.

Then I saw her squirm unconsciously. *Good,* I thought, *we have a chance.*

Kevin looked up, obviously happy to see another medic. "Breathing is irregular. Vital signs 160/40 BP, pulse rate 50. I can't tube her; every time I try she fights me."

Great another head injury! I knew we had to get an airway inserted in order to reduce the pressure caused by the blood pooling around her brain. Out on the streets the only way to do this would be to get a tube in her trachea and rapidly breathe for her. Without an adequate airway and thus appropriate oxygenation, she would probably die in surgery or, if she was lucky, live out her days as a vegetable.

"Let me give it a shot," I said. Kevin held her neck while I began to enter her mouth with the laryngoscope in an attempt to find her trachea.

I saw the vocal cords, a precursor of the windpipe, but when I went to pass the tube, the girl clamped down with her teeth. It was all I could do to get the laryngoscope out of her mouth.

I tried again and the result was the same. This time she moved wildly all over. *At least she was moving her arms and legs*, I thought. *She had something left up there.*

"Let's go, let's go," someone kept on saying.

I made the decision to stay: she would not live long without an airway. If we couldn't intubate her orally we would have to perform a cricothyrotomy. We would make an incision in the cricothyroid membrane in the neck and a shortened tube would be inserted directly into her trachea.

A lead medic for Riviera came over and stated they were ready to go. After speaking a moment, we both decided the boy would go by helicopter to Delray, while our girl would go to the closest facility, St. Mary's. He started to protest, initially, but I explained we had to get an airway in her and if it took a few minutes and she was flown to a further hospital, she might not make it. Grudgingly he agreed.

After Kevin prepped the equipment, we were ready to go. I had the most experience, so I decided to make the first cut.

Funny thing about the rules governing paramedics; we're not allowed to diagnose a head cold, but we're expected to perform life-saving surgery in a moment's notice without a hitch.

Kevin found the appropriate landmarks. My hand shook as I gently began to slice the top layers of the skin above her trachea. It was a tanned olive, just like a Barbie's.

With the first incision she squirmed and moaned a little but with every subsequent cut she would make a more guttural sound. The deeper the cut, the deeper the sound and the more violently she squirmed.

Another Riviera rescue arrived with one of their medics explaining that there had been some mix-up in their dispatch office.

I nodded, knowing full well that this kind of thing happened everywhere and it certainly wasn't their fault- they work even harder than we do. But I didn't say anything; instead I moved on- it was our mess now.

I felt like a Nazi surgeon performing some illegal surgery. Normally we would sedate someone like this to either get the airway orally or, if that wasn't an option, to ease the pain of this operation. But I didn't carry any valium on my truck and Kevin's truck was gone. As good as Riviera Fire Department was, I sensed their medics didn't agree with this.

I winced as I made yet another cut and again she writhed

in pain.

Paramedics tend to maintain a state of professional empathy. Between the chaos created by patients, family members and bystanders, it's the only way to do our job and bring some order to an explosive situation. We take charge, identify with the patient and treat the patient with a kind of "non-emotion"- an "it didn't happen to me" philosophy. You can't show up and really feel for these people or you'd quit before you were thirty and never get the job done. During some of the scenes I've been on I have had to pretend the patient is a mannequin and not a person, because the realization that it was a person would've been too much.

A partner of mine laid it on the line for me once, when he saw I was getting upset at the scene of a drowned two-year-old. He whispered, "Real men don't cry or show emotion. Do your job. It's not your kid."

Her skin was tough and bled little. I had done this surgery three times before, twice successfully.

The movements of her extremities were now becoming more inward to the body. The pressure around her brain was intensifying.

My radio squawked. "Engine 5 to Command, the chopper is five minutes out." I needed to get to the landing zone and make sure everything went smoothly.

I made another cut. She squirmed and I dropped the scalpel on the pavement. "Get me another one," I growled. By moving she had made me cut too high.

Rescue 1, my downtown unit, had arrived and they quickly came over to help with the girl. I gave Kevin the new scalpel. "I'll be right back," I said.

I made my way 50 feet to the landing zone. The Captain of Engine 5 would actually land them and when they did, the Riviera crew would turn the boy over to the chopper medics for transport.

In the distance the "thump-thump" of the rotors could be heard and soon a small speck in the sky turned into a 500,000 pound helicopter hovering over the captain, producing a deafening roar and a small windstorm. He backed off and they put down. The Riviera Medics hustled the boy over on their stretcher and the exchange was made.

Two down, one to go. I raced back to the girl. When I got there I found Kevin attempting to place the tube into her neck. He had done a good job correcting my mistake, but something was wrong.

Now the girl's movements were less animated: a bad sign. I tried the tube myself, pushing the short, clear tube into her now paling skin. It would enter a little, but not pass. I used more force, but I could see that I was almost collapsing the trachea so I let up.

"The hole it must not be big enough," said the Lieutenant of Rescue 1.

"It should be," I said, taking a closer look. "But something's wrong. Let's make it bigger."

Kevin took the scalpel.

My radio squawked. "Engine 5 to command- the chopper has left."

I rotated my body to talk into my radio and bumped into a kid in shorts and a T-shirt who was looking over my shoulder. At first I thought it was an off-duty cop.

"Look, man," I said. "You gotta get back."

Kevin was now making more sweeping cuts to puncture the girl's trachea.

"Is she gonna be okay?" he asked.

"Who the-" I almost yelled. "We're doin' our best. You need to get back."

"But I think I'm hurt."

"Huh?'

"I was in the car with her. I think I'm hurt."

I'm sure my jaw dropped. "You were in the car- that car?" I pointed to the totaled two-door and he nodded. "Well, let's sit you down and get a look at you." I waved some Riviera Fire-medics over to us.

"Where do ya hurt?'

"My elbow," he said, bending it back and forth. I could

tell he was stunned by all this activity.

"Is that all? No neck pain or anything?"

He shook his head. As he did this, a multitude of medically trained hands began to slap equipment on him, poke and prod.

I turned back to the girl. She was hardly moving now. Kevin was still cutting. "All right, Kev—let's try the tube once more and if it doesn't go, then just do the best to ventilate her on the way in to St. Mary's. You'll ride in with Riviera." Their truck was closest and already heading in the direction of the trauma center.

I put my hand on his shoulder. "We did the best we could."

Tired and disappointed, I turned back to the boy. Draped with equipment and injured arm in a sling, he was obviously at a loss for words. The medics gave me "thumbs up", signifying he was okay.

"Hey," I said. "Why aren't you hurt worse?"

"The seatbelt," he said.

"What? What?" I repeated. A news helicopter was now fluttering above us so I could barely hear.

"The seatbelt. I had it on; the others didn't."

I turned back to Kevin. Once again he was trying to insert the tube. It seemed to get held up and then finally it passed into the right position. "I got it!" he yelled.

He taped it down and attached the Ambu bag. "Now," I said. "Let's hyperventilate like crazy." Almost immediately she began to move around again, so much so we had to restrain her hands when we placed her on a backboard and then on a stretcher.

I took it as a good sign. Not a great sign but a good sign.

As we closed the doors of the Riviera truck, I told Kevin he'd done a good job. His shirt was soaked with sweat and his sunglasses were fogged over from the humidity. He smiled for the first time.

Someone tapped me on the shoulder.

It was the boy again. "Is- is she gonna be okay?" He was

obviously upset.

I looked at him for what seemed like an eternity. I wanted to tell him I was sorry for yelling; I wanted to explain to him the intricacies and fickleness of the traumatic head injury; I wanted to lecture him and be sure he knew how this could all have been avoided; and, most of all, I wanted to hug him and tell him everything would be okay. But I couldn't.

I put on my professional mask and turned, watching the rescue truck pull away. "We did our best. She needs a surgeon now."

Walking back to my truck I asked dispatch about our on-scene time.

"Eighteen minutes," was the reply. I swore under my breath.

* * *

I am staring at myself in the mirror when I come back to reality. I am no longer on scene.

I look down at my watch. Like some alien encounter in a B-movie, I realize I've lost 15 minutes. It's now closer to 1:30.

I'm dry now but I continue toweling off, taking my time.

I called about the three kids just after dinner. They all died. The boy in the seatbelt was the only one to survive, walking out of St. Mary's ER after about an hour of tests.

Perhaps we should have just "swooped and scooped" and let the trauma surgeons worry about it instead of staying on scene with the girl so long. Maybe that would have made a difference.

My mind is still spinning and I have a headache. *Headache...head wound... traumatic head injury...kids in seatbelts...fast cars...my car, my wife, my kids...*

Thirty seconds later I am on the phone, waking up my wife, trying not to talk about the call on I-95.

Instead I am making my point over and over. "Just

promise me you won't even start the car without having Cory and Christina in their seatbelts."

"Okay, okay," she says. "Brent, is everything all right?"

I don't answer.

"Was it a call?' she asks.

I picture all three kids strewn across the six-laned Interstate. I see the girl's pupils, I smell her hair, I feel her skin...

"Brent, are you okay?"

I remain silent.

"Brent?"

I bite my lip. "REAL MEN DON'T CRY, REAL MEN DON'T CRY," I keep muttering to myself.

Savior

The call came in as a non-emergency transport from South County Mental Health to some hospital I'd never heard of down south. I want to say it was "Holy Cross", but I think that's just my memory playing tricks.

I do know all I really wanted that morning was to transport this nutcase quickly and get back to bed.

At 4 a.m., South County was eerily quiet. From the distance it reminded me of a mad professor's house where Frankenstein was created or the Wolfman was lurking.

Inside I expected maniacal screams, but instead there were about five patients sitting on a couch watching TV with occasional loud voices in the background.

The nurse escorted us to a room in the back.

"This is Mr. J – real name unknown," he said, opening the door. In the room was a pale, skinny, thirty-ish gentleman with shoulder-length hair and the beginnings of a beard. "He's yet to be properly processed and diagnosed, but we believe he's a paranoid schizophrenic. He showed up this morning; we just don't have room for him."

He stood up as if to greet me, but instead made a cross in the air with his hand.

"Bless you," he said.

"Oh yeah," said the nurse. "He thinks he's Jesus Christ." He was dressed in a hospital gown that hung on his body. His hair was oily and disheveled and the skin around his mouth was chapped and peeling, the latter being a classic sign of the mentally ill.

An orderly brought us the paperwork and the male nurse thumbed through it.

"Everything is in order," he said. "Oh, you might want to take these," he held up some wrist and ankle restraints. "He can get violent."

"Jesus has a temper?" I said. Mr. J. stood up again and made another cross.

My partner and I looked at each other with raised eyebrows. "Nah," I said. "We'll take our chances."

We got the paperwork and a few minutes later we were on the road.

In the back of the ambulance, I made him comfortable on the stretcher while he quoted the Bible and blessed me several times. "Are we going to Bethlehem?"

"Yeah, sure," I smiled. How many of these transports had I done—30? 40? There had been so many, I couldn't remember.

He spoke of helping mankind, of saving souls. I moved uncomfortably in my seat.

"I disturb you, don't I?" he finally said, speaking more normally as opposed to the theatrical tone he'd been using.

"Yeah," I nodded. " I guess 'cause I have my own reservations about my beliefs."

"At least you do believe," he added. "It seems so hard for people to believe now."

He turned and looked deeply into my eyes. I didn't blink, but I tensed, ready for anything.

"You're a decent man, but you're torn. Not only with your beliefs; you wonder if you're doing the right thing as in helping the ill, but you feel like you have to do it."

"How'd you know that?" I asked, but he had turned away. He was back into his original routine, theatrical voice and all.

A few minutes later, my partner yelled back that we were almost there.

"Bethlehem?"

"No," I said truthfully. "You're going to another mental facility."

He was quiet, staring straight ahead and in a normal voice he said, "They put people away because they act like someone who is good? What kind of world would do that?"

"I don't know. I'm sorry," I said.

His voice changed again. "I don't blame you and I forgive you. You've been kind."

A minute later we arrived.

"But maybe it's best maybe to talk to these people," I was saying, trying to rationalize this for him. My partner opened the back doors. Two orderlies in white were with him.

I stood Mr. J up to walk him out.

"Not here!" he yelled, looking out the back. He began to flail his arms. "Not again!" I tried to get his hands but he pushed me away.

That's when the orderlies pounced. "No! No!" he repeated. I helped restrain his legs and all four of us carried him inside. The fight eventually left him and he said nothing. He wouldn't even look at me.

Closing my eyes on the trip home, I found I couldn't sleep. Maybe all he wanted to be was be a good person, to be Christ-like. If the real Jesus Christ came down today, would modern medicine institutionalize him too?

It had been a while since I'd been to church or read the Bible, but I remembered those early days in Sunday school. Religion had been such a big part of my life then; now I rarely thought about it except on certain holidays. I guess I'm too busy. *That's funny*, I thought- *too busy to save yourself.*

I'd gotten into this business to be Christ-like as well. To save people's lives, to save children. And I found that you didn't save that many patients when you needed to. They didn't tell me that when I signed up.

The job is either extremely stressful and difficult like

when you're working to save a cardiac arrest, or very easy
like, when I'm just baby-sitting patients- Mr. J, for instance.
People use medics like they use religion, for anything they
need at the time until we're all used up.

A savior—that's what I wanted to be. I wondered if
Christ ever felt like giving up.

There's been so much pain I've already seen in my life:
grandparents who grieve because we pulled their grandchild
out of a pool and couldn't save him, teens who drink and
crash their cars dying in the process, babies who have
AIDS...

The streets are evil sometimes, with all the shootings and
stabbings and drug deals gone bad. Those people need to be
saved, but no one could save them.

I wanted to be a paramedic so I could save the world,
but I found out I couldn't, so instead I just try to make my
own world livable. I guess, by doing this, I'm trying to save
myself—save my own sanity.

I closed my eyes, thinking about Christ and saving children while drifting off to sleep, realizing I probably
wouldn't think of these things again until the next holiday.

The Princess

When we picked her up I thought she looked familiar. But when I knew her, she'd been youthful, healthy and full of life; now she looked old, emaciated, personifying Cancer.

"Hi," she said, trying to catch her breath. "I heard you were doin'...this...I thought I might...see you." She paused, concentrating on the nasal canula in her nose, inhaling deeply. "You probably don't even recognize me."

I was tempted to subtly look around the truck for the report, but I sensed this was important to her so instead I studied her face. The moment took me aback, but her face, even though now skeletal, was etched in my memory. That face transported me to a simpler time that I could never forget.

"Hello, Glenda," I said and she smiled. I'd known her for over ten years. We'd grown up together, summers only, at the same day camp- from the time we were in minor camp to senior camp until finally we were junior counselors, ourselves partially in charge.

In my mind I saw a muddied picture of boys on swing sets and girls playing jacks, chanting rhymes and singing songs.

"Though we're not quite seven,
What is most like Heaven?
It's the joy that's found
With your arms around,
Just the right somebody to love."

Day camp. It had been years since I'd even thought about that time in my life. I remembered those days all too well, and they always brought a smile to my face.

It was when life was just a game of hopscotch or soccer; a time when if you had a football in hand and a dollar in your pocket, everything was going your way. A time when secretly holding hands beneath a tree next to the lake was the most important thing in the world.

Glenda had been voted "Princess of the Camp" three years running, and I was her athlete. At eleven years old, she'd been my first kiss.

It was awkward- hell, I hadn't seen her in 13 years.

"It's sure been a while, " she said, breathing deeply. "How... have you been?"

Then, grabbing my hand and gritting her teeth she said, "Oh God- this hurts."

To see her in such pain was more than I could take. "Don't worry, Glen," I whispered. "I'll take care of you."

Contacting the hospital, I argued with the ER until I got orders for morphine. They were explicit, since she was already on her own pain meds, only 5 milligrams.

I gave it rapid IV push and the pain seemed to subside. She relaxed and we were able to reminisce about the good old days. Me—the athlete and Glenda, the princess.

It was a short ride to the hospital, but I got the rundown: she'd been married and and divorced with no kids. She'd known him in high school; it had only lasted a few years.

Three years ago she began to get sick. When the doctors decided it was Cancer, they operated to remove what they thought would be a small part of her stomach. When they opened her up, they found it had spread too far too fast, so they sewed her up and gave her six months.

That was two years ago, she said, and for the last eight months she'd been on radiation treatments with no changes, other than the fact she was getting worse.

The pain hit her again, this time leaving her writhing. I remembered what the ER had said, but didn't hesitate: I gave her the another 5 of morphine.

Glenda thanked me and kissed me on the cheek.

"You know, sometimes I think those were the happiest days of my life," I whispered. "Me, too," she said.

Glenda was my first kiss and I would be her last.

I learned about her death when I was back at the ER less than two hours later with another patient.

"Though we're not quite seven,
What is most like Heaven?
It's the joy that's found
With your arms around,
Just the right somebody to love."

Cancer: such a dirty word it's stated in hushed tones. Poor Glen. There had been so much she'd said she hadn't done, but there just wasn't enough time. I guess there never is.

I thought about her pain and I wondered if it's not just as painful to remain here on this Earth. Since I've hit twenty-eight, there have been at least five people I grew up with who have died: auto accidents, overdoses, drownings and finally Cancer.

Every time I hear about another it hurts a little bit more; it makes me feel little bit more mortal.

Poor Glen. I felt about a hundred years old and very tired. Would it not be easier if maybe I was the one to go? I mean, with the bills and all the daily, trivial problems we take so seriously- is it worth it?

Who would care if that had been me? I mean, is it I and not my job that makes a difference? Because I'm here in this life, does my participation make it a better world, or am I just another number, another spoke in the wheel?

Buttoning my jacket, I looked at the stars. I'd miss

Glenda. Something in me had died with her; I'd never look back on those days the same way again.

The stars were bright that morning at 3 a.m., seeming to light up the ER parking lot and sparkle off a nearby lake. Standing alone next to the truck, I heard a medical alarm sound over the portable radio in my back pocket. Another call for my unit. I'd been on seven since dinner and on one of the last ones a good friend of mine had died.

"Let's go," I hollered to my crew. It looked like it was gonna be a helluva night.

Food, Fire and the Coffeemaker

She was like a heavy burlap sack weighing me down. Sometimes just the turning of a corner would make me stumble and I would have to re-balance her weight. I could not believe how heavy the little old lady was, and I knew I had to move as fast as I could.

* * *

We'd arrived at the scene first. It had been called in as a general fire alarm at an adult living facility known for its number of false alarms.

The primary pumper was already on another call, so being the rescue truck at that station we had responded instead. We finished dressing out in our bunker gear, moving slow and lackadaisically, having just finished dinner.

I'd arrived with "nothing showing", but as we got to the front door I noticed the smell of smoke. I advised dispatch and the other pumper that was responding, but I figured it was no big deal- a dinner-time smell of smoke usually just meant a burned-up pot of food on the stove.

But as we entered the building the smell became stronger...

It was a place I usually got the coffee that started my day- my local neighborhood gas station. It was a little place that had a homey feel to it. Joyce, the ever-efficient cashier with dark hair and coffee-colored skin, was always so happy to greet me in my uniform.

She always asked the same question. "Save anybody lately, Chief?"

And I always tried to fill a few minutes of her busy morning with exciting tales of shootings, cardiac arrests and dramatic auto accidents. She'd stunned me a couple of times with her retention and insight. "You know," she mused one morning, "It seems like you save one and lose two then save one and lose two more. I don't think I like that battin' average."

* * *

Residents were now moving out of their rooms on the first floor. If there was a fire it had to be upstairs. Women with walkers and men with canes moved slowly past me, wanting to know what was going on.

I explained I didn't know yet, advised them to leave their doors open and begin evacuation of the building.

We made our way up the stairs passing more concerned senior citizens on their way down. "What's happening? What do we do?"

I gave the same advice, saying everything was okay and that we had everything under control, and like a cue in a bad B-movie that's when the lights went out.

I had only been on the job about three years, so it was extremely rare for me to be the Lieutenant in charge and, being on the rescue truck, even rarer for me to arrive first at a fire. This made me a little nervous and self-conscious, since I had less time on than some of those I was supervising.

We paused on the second floor, looking in just long enough to confirm there was only light smoke there as well. That narrowed it down to being the third and final floor.

The floor was set up with three corridors lined with rooms on each side, all of them intersecting the one main avenue which lead to the stairwell. Having been in this building on calls before I knew there was no back stairwell, so there was no other way out.

Since there were three on my truck, we each took a corridor. I had to yell over the squealing fire alarm, but I thought they understood. I took the most western one. Most of the doors were already open with no one inside, but a few were locked, causing me to shoulder them a little and break the lock or the jam to gain access. It had been extremely dark in the stairwell, but on the floors you could see several feet in front of your step. It was so much better I could even save my flashlight by turning it off.

As far I could tell most everyone was already out, the booming alarm and the heavy smell of smoke alerting them. I was relieved as I approached my last locked door. I could see that the one after this was open and presumably evacuated.

In fire school they taught you to feel the door with your hand for heat so you don't walk into a raging fire without any warning. This door seemed cool, the wood finish rough against the back of my hand. I tried the handle and once again it was locked. I twisted the knob to the left and wedged a shoulder into the crack of the door and it popped open appropriately. I knew I had the right room as black smoke churned and glided toward the new opening. I covered my mouth. In the middle of the room I thought I saw something on the floor. Something familiar, something I should know.

In training they stressed that the most important action in any structure fire was rescue. You should determine in your initial size-up of the scene an estimation of the occupancy of the building, the number of victims threatened by fire and the easiest way to access and remove them.

Sometimes removal was accomplished through fairly complex alternate routes, like ladder trucks or fire escapes, and sometimes it was as simple as dragging them out the front door.

When I first found her she'd been on her side and barely conscious. The smoke was coming from the kitchen and I could see flames beginning to hop from somewhere in there to a curtain in the living room. I hefted her onto my shoulder and began to make my way to safety. Before I left I thought I heard a clank- again it was something I thought I should know—but I gave it no heed and didn't even look back.

Eventually I had her in a classic fireman's carry and she seemed to teeter with my every movement. Balancing her I moved back toward the stairwell yelling for my crew. The smoke was now thicker in the corridor and it stung my eyes. The alarm was so deafening it took me three yells before I heard my partners answer back. Eventually two bulky shadows made their way toward me.

I hacked through the smoke, "I gotta get her outa here. Tell dispatch the fire's on this floor down the western corridor. They'll need a line. Hook up to your air and make sure everyone's outa here. The only one I didn't get to was the very last door. The one south of the fire. Check it out and then get outa here. Don't take too long."

I was still hacking as I turned the corner, and with one final clearing cough I moved toward the stairwell. Funny thing about emergency situations: you have so much adrenaline going, it gets hard to keep some things straight, even for those of us who encounter them all the time. I had been to hundreds of serious auto accidents and cardiac arrests, but since I'd been to so many I'd grown accustomed to that kind of chaos. I never raised my voice; I never got confused.

How many high-rise fires had I been to? Five, maybe, so it was all still new.

I thought about putting her down and hooking up my airpack. But I decided against it, thinking I'd have her out in the fresh air soon enough.

My eyes were dripping as I pushed my way through the latched exit door to the stairwell. This was fresh, cool air compared to what I'd just been through. I sighed and rehoisted my prize. If I moved quickly I could be out of this mess in two minutes.

I started doing my balancing act down the stairs, every once in a while noticing a barely audible groan from my shouldered package. In the dark I had to feel my way down the stairs, pressing my left hand against the stuccoed walls. A strange thought crossed my mind that this didn't seem to be the same stairwell. It grabbed me and gave me goose bumps like ice cold rain on a summer's night. I shrugged it off though, since I knew there was only one.

I fumbled to get my flashlight. It wasn't in my left pocket or my right. Then I remembered the clank I had heard while leaving her apartment. I didn't panic; this was simple. We'd been up three stories, thus I should go down six sets of stairs to get to the first floor and out. *It's just a kid's game*, I said to myself, *known as blindman's bluff.*

Carefully I made my way down the six flights with each new step a mystery. After the initial set I turned my body sideways so I would not lose my balance when I went from landing to first step. I learned each stairway had ten steps while each landing was four big steps and four smaller ones. It seemed to take forever and then finally I found myself feeling for the first floor door. It pushed open easily and I began to pick up my pace, sensing I was almost out. I was still in complete darkness, but I knew if I moved down the corridor I would eventually find a handrail and then be able to see from the light coming through the front windows.

But all I could see was black. I didn't think it had been that dark before.

My left hand was outstretched for obstacles and familiar objects like the doors of the apartments which should have been on either side of me. What I didn't want to do was catch an open door square in the face. I kicked something and it moved easily, sliding on the floor. I carefully squatted down touching it. It was a cardboard box, and next to it another one. Why would boxes be out? I turned and walked ten steps to my right. Reaching out I felt nothing but air. Where the hell were the rooms?

I stopped. The corridor couldn't have been more than 5 or 6 feet wide.

Then, like an invisible door, it hit me. This place had a basement, didn't it? One for storage, only a half flight down. I must have miscounted and missed the first floor by one staircase.

The smoke was lighter down here, but I knew that if it

took a long time to put out the fire it could get a lot worse for us down there. It had already seemed like an eternity since I'd arrived with nothing showing.

I calmed myself, taking one knee to hook my mask to my airpack. The old lady hadn't made any sound in a while and now with this new turn of events I was worried for both of us. By feel I pushed the mask right and upwards and held it on her face, hooking the straps around her ears.

I stayed there for a moment to gather my thoughts. I had to find the stairwell again and go up one length of stairs and get out as soon as possible.

My right shoulder and arm were numb from her weight and I could feel I was sweating uncontrollably under my bunker coat. I stopped right where I was and turned to my left and walked ten steps back. I counted out loud.

I turned left again. *This should put me right in front of the door*, I thought. Pressing forward with outstretched hands, I came to something immovable. It was not a wall but some stacked crates or boxes. I figured I was too far left so I began sliding my left side against boxes to the right. This kept me in contact with the wall and dissipated some of her weight. My legs were now beginning to cramp so I leaned heavy.

After five steps I stopped. I now had another wall- a wall heading right as far as I could feel.

Where was that door? In my mind I went back over what I'd done. *Had I turned* left or right upon coming back to the wall? I'd made all left hand turns. Should there have been a right?

The lady was definitely not moving and I noticed my air mask had slipped off her face and was now dangling behind me like a tail. *Let it hang*, I thought, *I don't have time* for that now.

I took five more steps to the right: more boxes, no door- I'd gone the wrong way.

I started back left, totally confused.

Then I heard them: footsteps, muffled voices, banging equipment. I stopped. Where was it? I sensed to my left. I hurried, sliding my right hand against the wall and boxes. The noises appeared closer.

I knew those voices. I kept going. A wall then boxes; in, then back out. The voices were loud now. What's this- something different? I pushed with my whole body and sud- denly I was somewhere else. Fresher, cooler air. Made me realize I was back in the stairwell again.

I dropped to my knees breathing heavily. The voices were trailing off. "Hey, help me! Hey, gimme a hand!"

The voices began to come back. "Who? What?"

"The stairwell- help- I gotta lady-"

Soon familiar gloved hands took her from me. The lack of weight was relieving, almost intoxicating. I was helped up. Wobbly, I made my way through the lobby on my own. Dusk was the color of pewter through the front windows, but it seemed like high noon to me. I worked my arm and squeezed my neck in an attempt to get my nerves feeling again.

When I got outside I went back down on my knees, struggling to get my airpack off and then my coat. More friendly hands helped me, cups of water were shoved in my face.

"Fire's out," somebody said. "Everybody's evacuated."

I shook with dehydration and tried to catch my breath.

Just to my right four medics worked fervently on my gray-haired lady. As I listened, I winced. "Thready pulse- respirations severely labored-"

It was my fault.

The Battalion Chief knelt in front of me. "We were ex- pecting you 15 minutes ago."

"I got lost." I tried to get up, but my legs wouldn't work.

"You run outa air?"

"No," I said, feeling foolish. "I didn't hook up until the end, then I put the air mask on her."

The BC paused, his old eyes looking me over. "Yeah, first they said saccharin could give ya cancer, then it was bacon. I wonder what they say about going into burning buildings."

I nodded, point well taken. *Use your airpack, idiot.*

"I'm ventilating her," said the medic at her head as he squeezed much needed oxygen into her lungs through a mask.

I couldn't help, so instead I got religious. "Please God," I prayed. "Not because of me."

Normally if I'd made a mistake on a medical call I'd really beat myself up. Hell, I should be good at those, I figured, they were 85% of our call volume. But it wasn't that way in a fire. I hadn't been to one yet that'd been mistake-free. They were too physical and volatile, always changing. And they were so few and far between that regardless of training, it was difficult to reach any level of perfection.

I'd done my job; I'd gotten her out.

Then I heard the words that would make me feel invincible for two whole days.

"Her heart rate's up. Hey, she's breathing on her own and moving."

As I entered the gas station that next morning, Joyce gave me a sideways look as I prepared my morning coffee.

"Hey, Chief– you save anybody lately?"

And as I limped toward her I was all smiles. "Have I got a story for you today...."

Sunday Drive

I knocked on the door expecting no answer.

Maybe I knocked too lightly; maybe I didn't want her to come to the door. Slowly I turned, figuring that I'd given it my best shot.

Then I heard the screen door creak open. "Yes?" she said. She was in her fifties, I imagined, different than what I had remembered.

"Yeah," I began. I was not prepared for this.

"Ma'am, I'm sorry to bother you, but I was one of the paramedics to respond to that accident that happened out on the corner a coupla months back. You know the accident?"

She said nothing but instead eyed me warily. Finally she broke the stare. "Come in, please."

I sat across from her on a brightly colored, well-maintained couch. A table sparse with magazines separated us. "Can I get you some coffee?" she asked.

I almost said "yes" to procrastinate more, but instead shook my head "no."

"So?" she began, not willing to give an inch or make it easy on me.

"Yeah, I was on the rescue truck that responded when your son died—I was in charge—I just wanted to say I was sorry." The statement hung in the air like cigar smoke in a crowded bar.

There, I said it. Time to go.

She picked her words carefully. "You waited six months to come tell me this?"

I nodded, rubbing my hands together. I was very un-comfortable.

Again there was silence, the ticking of a clock the only sound.

I had not wanted to think of the call; it all was too painful. An eighteen-year-old boy lying twisted and broken in the front seat, killed by one smack of a speeding, out-of-control vehicle as he turned onto the main road. They esti-mated the other car had been moving at 80 to 100 miles per hour.

I had crawled into the car by myself as he was curled un-der the dash with no pulse. The crowd around the vehicle was hysterical, begging us to work him, screaming at the he-roes. Our flashing lights illuminated their distraught faces. I left one of my partners there to preserve the scene and I ran with my second medic to the other car.

There was massive damage to the car and a fire in the en-gine compartment. We put that out and worked on getting the driver out of the car. She was forty and you could smell the alcohol on her breath from two feet away. Her legs had been crushed and rolled under by the dashboard.

It would take us nearly 30 minutes to get her out, but we would eventually prevail and save her life. I'd feel strange about it from that moment on.

"We were just sitting here when we heard the accident," she said. "And we ran out knowing he'd just left-"

"I know," I interrupted. "I saw you."

"And we begged you to save him and help him, but you did neither."

"Ma'am, he was already gone. In blunt trauma the save rate is zero when they're killed instantly like that. I'm sorry."

"And instead you saved the lady, that drunken woman who hit him."

"Yes." I nodded, looking down. Why did I come here? What was I trying to prove?

"And now you want absolution? Well, damn you! Damn you! You should have been there for my boy!"

Her face was twisted and knotted in a grotesque mask of anger.

"I will not forgive you! Never!"

"I'm not asking you to," I said. "I just feel badly for you."

"Six months later you feel badly- or guilty?"

I looked up. "I shouldn't have come."

"Then go! You call yourselves lifesavers, and you don't even-" She put her hands to her face, but she wasn't crying.

I stood up, speaking with force. "Look, this was a bad idea- I did nothing wrong that night. There was nothing I could do. I just wanted to say that I'm sorry for your loss."

She was looking off into the distance, hands in her lap. "Go," she said. "Just go." Then she added, "We loved him so. He was our only- his father is lost now."

I began to make my way toward the door, hands stuffed in my pockets.

Upon reaching it, I looked back. "I apologize for coming this morning. It was a bad idea."

There was no reply, so I continued outside. Seconds later I felt her presence behind me at the screen door. I turned halfway around. "Look," she said. "I know there was nothing you could do. I'm sorry for treating you that way."

I nodded. "It's okay; I'm getting used to it."

"You help people and that's good," she said, "but I think overall you've got a shitty job." I nodded and moved to my car.

I still remember her at the screen door, unmoving and frozen in time. Maybe she was reliving one of his birthday parties, a baseball victory or an exceptional report card. Perhaps she'd stay that way for an hour or more; quite possibly, these memories were the only peace she had nowadays. Maybe she could never watch a sunset, read a book again, or do anything for that matter without thinking of him.

But if I'd done nothing wrong then why did I feel so badly? After that, I just recall speeding away in my Camaro, repeating over and over those words which had stung the worst and rang of the most truth: "You've got a shitty job."

Advice From A Bare-Breasted Dancer

It's strange: everything seems to be rolling along all right and then you wake up one morning and someone you love is dead, gone forever. And class, this brings us to our next equation: the death of a loved one = one blubbering out-of-control fire-medic.

So I sat there at the bar, staring at my drink. He was only sixty-eight-years-old, with no cardiac history and as healthy as anyone I knew.

"You know, *I* lost my father once," said a voice next to me. "I know what you're going through."

It took me a minute to focus on the voluptuous, bare-breasted dancer I had just given a dollar to. I wasn't sure what she wanted: maybe another dollar, maybe my entire wallet.

"Huh?" I managed.

"I said, 'I lost my father once', too," she reiterated. I particularly liked the "once" part. I was tempted to ask, "How many daddies you got, hon?"

She went on. "The best I can tell you is that life goes on. I'm sure your father wouldn't want you sitting around sulking, especially *here*!"

Questions raced through my head as I looked over this sweaty, buxom, perfume-soaked, farm animal-like dancer. Questions like: Where was *here*, anyway, and does the management know you're giving advice like this?

Instead I opted for saying "Huh?" again.

"I said," said the dancer, now red in the face and out of breath from both dancing and yelling. "Life goes on. It's up to you to keep his memory alive!"

Alive. Yeah, I remembered my dad when he was alive. He'd been a staunch, aristocratic businessman from a long line of businessmen. And now all that history...all his stories, his views and his opinions were gone.

I lost my mother at eighteen, my grandparents at twenty-two and finally my father at twenty-eight. They were all gone—all my advisors.

But my dad was the only one who'd been truly healthy, and then- BANG! He dies overseas from a massive heart attack while traveling 2000 miles away. This is while I sat here in South Florida with all this training, considered by some to be the best in my field, and I couldn't help him. I save strangers everyday, but I didn't have a chance to save my own blood. There was some laughable irony there somewhere, but I wasn't in the mood for either the searching of it or the comedy itself.

"—but I found out that keeping busy was the only way to get over it-"

Oh my God, I thought. *She was still there and still talking!*

Hell, he wasn't perfect, but who is? He did the best he could raising me, but I didn't really even know him then. I got to know him as an adult and I liked him not only as a father but also as a friend.

"—that was in '82 and then I moved to-"

I was really hoping some ex-cowboy would happen by and mistake her for a fair-sized sow and hog-tie her in 12-15 seconds for a new bar record.

Now, I'd give a dollar to see that, I thought.

He seemed to do everything right for all the right reasons. He went to war, ran his own business, retired at forty-five, and when my Mom got chronically ill, stayed with us, remaining totally faithful.

You don't hear of too many people like that in today's day and age. Hell, I wish I had those kinds of morals!

"—but you must keep his memory alive through your children and your grandchildren-"

That was scary. The bare-breasted dancer was beginning to make sense. That reason, and the fact that the bartender had cut me off because I'd asked for a "Tin and Gonic" 3 times and a "Grin and Bubonic" twice, made me decide it was definitely time to go.

The sun was setting and there was a slight South Florida drizzle in the air.

Great. A Perfect end to a perfect couple of days.

I asked the bouncer to call me a cab and like most aspiring young, out-of-work comics he said, "You're a cab- now get going." I didn't even crack a smile and he asked me what was wrong.

I simply replied, "I buried my father this week."

"Oh," he said, almost running to the phone.

Memories flooded my mind while I waited for the cab. There was my brother and I hurrying to decorate his birthday cake before he got home, arguing the entire time how each of us knew he liked it; making a peanut butter and jelly sandwich with his help for Santa Claus on Christmas Eve: his stories of business, of college and of World War II; of places he'd traveled; his recollection of great football games–his whole life.

Taking his obituary out of my pocket, I studied it. Ten lines could sum up a man's whole life. It wasn't fair. Then it came to me: if the memories were kept alive, he would still be alive in all of us. The bare-breasted dancer *had* been right. It *was* up to us, up to me.

It was a long drive home.

My dad once said if you can look at yourself in the mirror and be happy with the kind of man you see in the reflection, then you've done all right with your life. Opening up my wallet, I took out his picture.

Someday, I thought. *I hope to look in the mirror and see the kind of man my father was and then maybe I'll have some peace.*

Resting my head on the front seat, I thought of mothers, fathers and grandparents and my most precious memories of growing up until reluctantly I fell asleep.

Bigger and Better Things

I never knew exactly where he was coming from, but I knew he was not medic material.

It was obvious from the first time he said, "It wouldn't be so bad on the medic truck if we didn't have to go to all those sick people." It was at moments like this that I knew he was destined for something else, something greater than EMS.

I only worked with John Palmer (not his real name) nine or ten times, but he was constantly coming up with little insights into his character. Out of those nine or ten times, for instance, it only took about three for him to figure out how to fill out that "complicated" trauma form fairly correctly. Still, on one shift he wrote five reports before realizing he wasn't using black ink. That particular shift was a long 24 hours.

It was on that same shift that I found John, who was always concerned with money, rolling pennies he'd found in his car. With a straight face (the man had no sense of humor) he said, "You know those penny rollers are great, but they sure make a big bulge in your pocket, and it's a bear to open them to get the right change."

Then there was John on politics: "I think President Carter should give more tax breaks to the rich." He said this proudly one Sunday; I didn't have the heart to tell him that had been two presidents ago.

We eventually termed these out-of-whack statements as *Palmerisms.*

And then there was the day after a big night out when he expounded, "Thirty dollars for tickets, fifty for dinner, ten for gas- I don't know where all my money goes."

But it was one day while we were in the local 7-11 that I realized he had to be destined for other things. After picking up a $100,000 candy bar, he said with his usual straight face, "I love these things and they are always on sale. And I gotta be careful 'cause I don't know where my money goes anyway."

Enough was enough. "You know, John," I said earnestly. "You should be in administration or something-maybe a city manager."

At twenty-seven, tall and lanky and always with an olive tan, John often bragged about being a lifeguard at one time. My question to him was, "Exactly how much sun did you get?"

Not surprisingly he was one of the people to see Elvis alive and well at a Wal-mart. And when he would talk about the rescue "rut" he was in and solutions to it, he'd always end with something like, "Oh well, at least it might break up the monopoly."

Needless to say, I wasn't the only one to study his medic license for authenticity- me and about three quarters of the other employees.

He wasn't a bad medic (just so long as he didn't touch me), but there were certain concepts he had a hard time grasping, for example on shooting calls he would usually cut through the bullet holes in a shirt to expose the patient's chest. This totally destroys physical evidence for the police. He could never remember that; I guess he figured it was a lot easier using a hole already there than making one with scissors.

And if the patient was shot in the arm, that was where he'd put the IV. I would always say the same thing: "John, if we do that, won't all the fluid we put in him run out the hole?" Common sense, eh? Oh, don't get me wrong–John could get complicated theories. It seemed to be the simple ones he had a hard time with.

Like the fact when we were out of the truck, we had to have the portable radio with us *and* turn it on to hear any calls.

But overall, I enjoyed my time with John Palmer and what I'd foreseen eventually came true. He retired after his one year anniversary to go on to bigger and better things to which he was far more suited.

Now years later, as I drive down main boulevards, I have to smile: there's John on a billboard, smiling back at me. "RE-ELECT JOHN PALMER TO THE STATE SENATE" the billboard reads. "HE'S A MAN YOU CAN UNDERSTAND."

Yeah, good old John- better him up there in Tallahassee with them, I always think, then here with us.

Wishing the Time Back

It wasn't that my father wasn't a good man or that I wasn't a good son, but sometimes it seems like all it takes is a career and some time away to create a ravine in a relationship.

I don't even remember when we stopped being that close. Who knows? What does it matter now, anyway?

It was cut-and-dry back then: I didn't have time.

We spoke on the phone, but it was the usual thirty-something work bullshit—nothing too personal, of course; it was always conveniently distant. Now I realize it should have been much more than that.

I was always too busy for drinks by the pool.

Who would have thought he'd die at such a young age? I'd always thought there would be more time to be together.

Time to say "I love you." That's my biggest regret. Ambition can be an awful thing, especially when it involves family.

I'll never forget the funeral. The heat was unbearable; the words from the speaker meaningless. At first I thought it was sweat running down my face, but it turned out to be tears.

Big macho fireman.

I just wish I could talk to him once more, just to tell him how I feel.

"Once more"—more meaningless words.

My son just turned three the other day and I can see his grand-dad in him. I tell him what I fine man he was, and I'll be damned if what happened between him and me will happen between my son and me.

I miss him, and I realize now it's my cross to bear.

Now I take all relationships seriously. I am never too busy to see an old friend or play a game with my son.

Five years is a long time. And as much as you wish, you can't get time back.

So, there I sit, cradling my son in my arms, talking to him like I wish I'd spoken to my father years ago.

Pretty Maids

They come in the early morning as sparrows, swooning down over my bed. They watch me sleep and dream. They chirp only on occasion, content, so that my peace is restful. Slowly, though, they begin to turn. Their slight black wings sprout tufts of gray feathers too large for their bodies. Their beaks become massive and hooked; their nails are now talons.

I begin to wake; I know they are here.

They have come to finish my liver off, to digest the beginnings of cirrhosis. They have come to blind me for the things I've seen. They guffaw at my failures.

They circle once more.

I am fully awake now. The re-taste of gin and bourbon is warm in my mouth by way of my esophagus.

Once more around and they are smiling. There are just two of them, but they are formidable and fierce. There is no defense. Maybe, I hope, they will leave this time.

They swoop up to the ceiling. They are ready and I cover my head with a pillow.

They come at me and I feel nothing but the poking of the pillow. I close my eyes but still see nothing but dead bodies...

I find myself in the bathroom, my head in a sink full of water. My eyes are red and puffy; my head pounds. My mouth is dry like sand.

Some drunks fall off the wagon while some are thrown from a speeding vehicle.

I'm not your typical drunk (I guess we all aren't), I can drink beer but not the hard stuff.

I examine the mirror, a ritual for the drunk. Do I have any scars, any black eyes?

What did I do, exactly? What set me off?

Oh, I forgot to tell you. I drink because of my work; that much I've rationalized. Firefighter-paramedics always drink because of their work. Whether it's from too much time off or the things they've seen, both are pretty good reasons.

The term firefighter-paramedic really doesn't explain what we do. We are the "illusion" of safety and medical aid. It is the same for the police department, they are the "illusion" of legal representation and security in any society. Primarily, we are the drive-by doctor of the poor and the homeless, those people whom the middle class don't want to know exist. They stab or shoot each other over drugs, or they contract AIDS and TB.

They die lonely deaths which accountants, pharmacists and suburban moms will never hear about except for maybe a quick fifteen seconds on the evening news. They unload their frustration and angst against the establishment on us. We bear that onus.

The first cup of coffee is the most difficult. You don't want to keep it down. You may even straddle the porcelain deity for strength. Guilt kicks in as your mind plays the night back to you in a piecemeal fashion.

The second and third cup go down easier, then maybe something for the pain. Two Tylenol each morning: a drunkard's best friend.

I think the best quote about drinking is one from a movie: "Not everybody drinks because they are poets. Some of us drink because we're not poets." Fortunately, I am a poet—I attempt to account for my life's actions on paper. It seems to give my failures meaning and when written it hurts less, but I don't drink because I'm a writer or because I have some base sense of creativity or empathy. I drink because it makes me forget the calls I've been on. It brings up further crises with which need to be dealt and the former event is lessened.

I check my watch and find out it is early. Now I realize I am tired. Passing out is not restful; it is necessary. I toy with the idea of calling in sick: an act with which I never follow through. Going to work this way is part of the punishment.

When you've been a fire-medic long enough and seen enough, you tend to not want to experience certain things again, it makes the work distasteful. Two teens en route to prom are T-boned by a drunken Jehovah's witness and killed instantly. Their bodies are pummeled and broken; necks, arms and legs are at totally wrong angles. You can hear the broken bone ends rubbing against each other as you move them.

These are the scenes you hope to never see again. These are the ones which makes every auto accident you roll on for months become a test of your strength. These are the memories which make you hold your breath and clench your teeth every time you think about work.

But it wasn't that that set me off this time.

I glance up at the phone, hoping it will ring with someone on the other line spouting, "Hey Braunworth, you don't have to come in today- is that okay?"

The phone is smudged from use and covered with those 3 numbers which call me to work each shift. 911... 911... 911...

I know now what set me off. It comes back to me in a sweaty flash of sobriety. I wasn't sure what was real or not before, but I do now.

It was something I volunteered to do on my day off: talk to a second grade class about fire safety and first aid. Maybe it's not exactly what I would normally want to do on my off day, but I didn't mind. You have to keep giving to the community; it's good PR and I've always liked dealing with kids. So when I was asked by the Fire Bureau I said no problem.

I gave my little speel about not smoking, wearing your seatbelt and not talking to strangers and had just started to start on the Stop, Drop and Roll lecture when, as usual, I was bombarded by questions.

"Have you ever been in a fire?" "Have you almost ever died?" "Have you ever seen a dead body?"

Yes, yes and yes. Then I gave a brief diplomatic and politically correct explanation of each. Fires aren't fun...Yes, I've almost died, but that's what I get paid for...Sometimes, unfortunately, I see dead people or people about to die and then I try to save them. It's very sad sometimes.

The pretty blond teacher cracked her whip and told them no more questions until the end. That lasted for another seven, maybe eight minutes.

I spoke of how firefighters dress in a fire, how we look like some scary monster and sound like Darth Vader, but if you see us or hear us and you're hiding during a fire you need to either come to us or call out.

Question and answer time again. "Are fires really hot?" "I had a friend who got burned in a fire." "One time I was in a car wreck and had to go to the doctor—did you take me?"

Yes, they are. That's why you need to stay low... Sorry about your friend... I dunno; I might've taken you.

"Now, class," said the pretty blond. "Let's let him speak and save these for the end."

"It's okay," I mused. "I'm about done anyway." They were only second graders.

"Do you ever drive the truck?" "Can you tell if somebody's heart is good?" "Have you ever seen any kids burned up?"

With all the emotional baggage we carry, it's hard to know when something somebody might say could trigger a response. I've saved patients and seen patients die right in front of me, and didn't give it a thought until somebody did something or said something that reminded me of it. Sometimes it was a good response; sometimes not so good.

The event came rushing through my mind like a tidal wave...

I was just getting off duty and swung by central station for some administrative reason, not that I truly do anything administrative on a regular basis: it's rare. I'm a lieutenant on a rescue truck. Usually the rank of Lieutenant dictates a certain separation from the troops, but at my fire department there is none. You're one of three on the truck. You're the boss of the unit- king of the grunts. You make all the decisions and when the shit hits the fan it's your ass on the line.

Normally, I tried not to do these types of things on my off days, but we'd had a good night with only one call, a cardiac arrest with which we shocked, on the second defibrillation, back to life. Like Jesus with Lazarus, her pulse began to bound and breathing, at first irregular, began to level off as did ours. So, I was feeling pretty good about my job, myself, and life in general.

But for whatever reason I was downtown working on some meaningless project for some meaningless committee I was assigned to since I was "an officer."

I was shooting the breeze with the men about sports and calls in the bay when the dispatcher came across. "Engine 3, Rescue 3, Engine 1A, Engine 1B respond to a structure fire with persons trapped."

The dispatcher blurted out the garbled address- one in zone 3, the north end of town.

"Additional information," she added. "There are three children trapped in the structure."

The men slid the pole, donned their fire gear and left in professional fashion, air horns blaring and sirens wailing down the road.

My heart lept as I watched the big engines roll away. I had never heard of a call being dispatched as anything but a "possible this or a possible that," and usually we never got information about somebody being trapped until we got there.

I remembered pulling a lady out of a window in just my bunker pants one fire. I decided not to dress due to her screaming so much, as there was no way to ignore her and get ready. After I pulled her out hacking from a window, she told me her baby was inside. I didn't inquire further; I told the responding engine, got ready and waited. When we got inside we searched while others doused the stove fire with water. We found no crib or baby's room, only a poodle on her last leg. "Baby" survived and the woman was estatic.

Consequently, I was concerned, but I figured that John Q. Citizen certainly can exaggerate when he calls 911. How many shootings had I been to that turned out to be false alarms? How many assaults had I been to when not only was the victim shot but we were getting the patient history and background from the shooter?

It was probably nothing, I figured, but I kept within ear-shot of a radio speaker.

Engine 3 arrived with heavy fire showing. The Captain told Engine 1B to make the hydrant and Rescue 3 to get ready for a primary search, the initial search made for viable victims.

The Battalion Chief arrived taking command of the situation.

Rescue 3 came back. "She says the bedroom. We have serious flames."

Minutes went by. Engine 1 came on the radio. "Fire's out. We're going in."

Another minute passed. "The search," said the Chief. "How 'bout the search?"

No one replied, then a moment later, I heard, "Chief, this is Rescue 3. We have three Code 10's. No patients. Better call the Bureau for an Inspector."

There was an unearthly silence on the radio, like the

pause after an emergency broadcast test. Perhaps everyone was saying a prayer.

I knew what had happened: A Code 10 was radio talk for a fire death. With this knowledge, I hung my head and slid the pole on my way to the scene.

Never in my life had I seen a worse looking fire incident. A line of neighbors looked on, shaking their heads, watching the mother cry and scream at the top of her lungs with a poor driver-engineer attempting to calm her and keep her from re-entering the building. All the other firefighters busied themselves, a sure sign that something had gone awry. One firefighter-paramedic I knew fairly well was sitting on the tailboard of the pumper, silently crying. I could see a newly-formed patch of redness on the back of his neck. I wasn't going to ask, but I suspected he had tried to make entry on his own without waiting for water.

My suspicions were confirmed as I looked at the house: the bedroom they spoke of was charred from the window sill to the ceiling inside.

An Inspector was already at the door scribbling notes. I nodded to him questionably that I was wanting to go inside. He nodded back. "It looks like the kids were playing with matches while the mother was doing dishes. She noticed smoke. She said she only left them alone for a few minutes. The fire was too much for her or our guys. It's not pretty."

There is a point when you don't want to see anymore pain, especially when you're not on duty, but I was there and I could not fathom that an entire family of children could be gone so quickly. I guess I had to see for myself.

They were in the closet- pretty maids all in a row- leaning on top of one another. The first one was about four-years-old, then six maybe and then the older one, maybe eight, give or take a year. It looked like you could reach out and shake a shoulder and wake them all up, but when you got closer you could feel the heat from them and notice just the slightest bit of blistering on the outside side of the outside kids.

God bless the children and have pity on the firemen, I thought. *We're just men and women trying to help and we have to see these things.*

The mother was now in the house and I could hear her cries and whimpers. Three children—you feed them and teach them to walk and dress, play tag with them, go to school plays, drive them to baseball games and do homework with them and one day they're gone.

Parents should never be asked to bury their children. It's not fair. You put such energy into raising them and caring for them so that they can have a better life.

Outside I said nothing to anyone. Nothing could be said; only things you'd later regret.

I could hear some of the men, though; in hushed tones, a few swore they'd quit. Others spoke about being unable to get to them from the window. Their voices warbled as the reality set in. No one smiled, and no one liked their job that day.

I left there feeling sick to my stomach and I was ill for two days. It's not like I thought about it all the time; maybe my body just decided that after seeing three dead kids that this was as good a time as any to give into sickness.

I didn't get drunk and I didn't cry.

* * *

The class was silent when I didn't answer right away.

I sat there saying, "Yeah, I've...ah...seen...ah...some ...kids...yeah...I've...ah seen...some...ah...kids..." Over and over. My eyes must have misted up pretty good, because by the time I got to my car my right shirt sleeve was damp from wiping my face.

I remember stumbling through the halls, still babbling. Teachers and kids were looking at me like I was a mental patient.

The blonde teacher walked me out.

"Hey," she said. "I don't know what happened with those kids, but if you ever need to talk."

A scribbled number on a card was handed to me.

All I could manage was a "ah...thanks...ah...yeah...ah." I felt as foolish as anyone driving away. The firefighter came to help the kids and they decided he needed help.

In my book there's only one way to cure foolishness: forget about it. So I stopped at the closest bar. I started with a shot of tequila and followed that with four Jack and cokes. That was just the first stop.

The rest is history, as they say.

Well, I *didn't* go to work that day: I called in sick. I guess I was done punishing myself. I did sit around feeling sorry for myself the entire morning, then I finally made an appointment with an Employee Assistance counselor, part of a city program designed to help cops and firefighters deal with psychological problems. We met at 1 p.m. and talked until about four. I explained it all. She told me I shouldn't feel so guilty about things which were beyond my control. I agreed and I vowed to stay off the hard stuff.

I picked up a six-pack and went by the beach to watch the sunset. When you've seen children die in fires and tried to help busted up near-dead teens in auto accidents, you have a tendency to feel that there is no God, or why would He do this to us? But in your heart you know there's a God and maybe you're not supposed to understand, but just to try to do your job and cope. No one ever said life had to be easy.

So I sat there and watched the sunset and had one beer thinking of all the lives I *had* saved. Maybe I took it all too seriously; maybe it was all an excuse to get drunk. No doubt I've been ruined in some ways by what I've seen, but there is good in life. There's got to be.

A little drizzle came along.

I was amazed at how bright and how different the colors were in a rainbow. It had been a while since I'd sat down and really looked at one. It was incredible. Finally, at about 8 p.m. I left for home, leaving the other five lukewarm beers resting lonely in their holder near an ocean shower, no doubt eagerly awaiting their next victim.

Bitter Tears

Holidays at the Fire Department have a long history of being slow starters, and that Easter Sunday was no exception. Although most everybody had had some kind of celebration the day before and the anticipation of seeing loved ones later in the day for dinner on duty was in the air, it was still hard to get it together and go check out those trucks. The fact that we were at one of the busiest stations in the entire county didn't help, either.

The lunch and dinner menus had been made, and since I was in charge of the medic truck that day it was up to me to get to the store and pick up the food before we got too busy.

I was at Station #3 located in the north end of the ghetto in West Palm Beach and just a stone's throw away from Riviera's "meaner streets", so I knew we should hurry up and go to the store before we began responding to assault after assault as our citizens began to drink more and more to celebrate this religious holiday.

There was a light banter around the station of what was done the night before and who would be coming to eat and visit that afternoon, as well as some stories from the married folk about "little Johnny" or "little Susie" and what cute things they'd done lately.

My second medic and I finished the monotonous task of the daily truck check about 8:45 AM. It was a "holiday routine"—another time-honored, firehouse tradition which meant only the most needed chores be done around the station. I still really don't know what that means since I've never really done anything on holidays but eat and run calls. We made our way to the store and let the other firefighters on the engine worry about what needed to be done.

After our shopping spree, which was surprisingly un-eventful, I settled in a chair to read the paper while the others began to prepare the first meal of the day.

Our first call came in at 10:30 AM as a possible shooting, which would probably surprise most anybody but those who live and work in West Palm Beach, Florida. I've often commented that it is the most incredible city I've ever known. It's the only city I've seen where one can view million-dollar homes along Lake Worth or dine in ostentatious wealth in a penthouse overlooking the rich and famous in Palm Beach, while only two blocks over, you have wooden shacks with crack dealers hovering out front, where robbery and death lurks in every corner.

It was like the beauty and the beast.

* * *

We arrived at the little house on 23rd Street to find about ten people out front, milling around and waving us over. They were all dressed extremely well as if they'd just come from church.

"What's up? What seems to be the problem?" I asked after I got out of the truck and proceeded to get our equipment.

This was definitely odd, since at most shootings there were usually people flailing their arms, crying or screaming. A robust, black gentleman answered back, shaking his head. "I think he's dead."

Upon entering the house, I saw it was decorated with a lot of religious paraphernalia, which was very typical for this part of town.

It seemed to be the kind of cluttered home you usually find with older people since they can't get around as well any more. Now some people say death sounds like Beethoven's Fifth Symphony, but I know the sound of death: it's the continuous humming of flies. Death has a smell and a taste for that matter, and it was definitely evident to me then that whoever was in the house was, in fact, dead and had been for some time.

I found him in the kitchen; I figured he was approximately seventy-five-years-old. He was lying on his back, eyes open and staring at the ceiling. It appeared that his throat had been cut and that he'd been stabbed in the mid-chest area. His face seemed all bloated and bruised as if he'd been beaten severely.

I quickly checked a pulse and then his leg joints to assure rigor mortis had set in so as not to disturb the body too much. Once I knew he'd been "down" a while and that we wouldn't be "working" on him, I secured the area and told dispatch to notify the detectives as well as a normal police unit, because I had a definite homicide.

I was so quick in doing this that my partners didn't even get into the kitchen before I'd sealed it off. I wanted minimal disturbance of the crime scene before the detectives got there.

While I waited for PD to arrive, I checked to see if the windows and doors were secure in an attempt to figure out if the killer had broken in or not. They were locked up tight and there seemed to be no signs of forcible entry.

The gas stove still had a burner lit with a charred pot of food on it. I turned it off and began to surmise that the killer almost had to be someone this man had known.

With the scene secure and my conclusions about what had taken place reached, I left the kitchen and the house to wait for the detectives outside. I learned that the people who had been standing in front of the house when I arrived had, in fact, come from church and that the deceased had been their Reverend. When he didn't show up for the Easter Sunday service, some of the members had become concerned and walked to his house, only to find him dead in the kitchen as I had.

When the detectives arrived, I welcomed them as if I were a dog waiting for his master. I explained what I did, why I did it and what I thought had happened.

After looking around themselves, the detectives agreed. It did appear, since there was no forced entry and due to the severity of the wounds, that the victim did know the killer and that he did not want the Reverend talking.

They complimented me and shook all of our hands so as to indicate that it was a job well done. We even had a laugh over the fact that when the call first came in, they began to head over here "just 'cause they had a feeling."

When we got to the station everyone seemed to be slapping me on the back and telling me I had hogged all the glory, the idea being that so many crime scenes are screwed up because when we get there we tend to mess up the entire area since we are usually only concerned with either calling a "dead on scene" or saving a life. Unfortunately, when we do that, we usually destroy many clues which could lead the police somewhere.

In between lunch and dinner we ran only a few calls, the assaults for a holiday totaling a lowly count of three or four.

We were even fairly slow until bedtime. As I lay in bed I thought of the day's events. I was still very proud of how I preserved that scene. I drifted off to sleep for maybe an hour and then I awoke sweating and coughing. I even thought that the alarm might have gone off for a call. When no one else stirred I figured I'd imagined it and ran to the bathroom, dousing my face with cool water. That's when I looked in the mirror.

What the hell was wrong with me? I thought. Today, Easter Sunday, I'd found a man- no not just a man, a Reverend, dead, murdered in his kitchen and I had no feelings about it. I mean I was happy about what I did on scene, but shouldn't I be upset, or at least somewhat bothered that a holy man was killed on the holiest of days?

But I felt nothing like that. *My God,* I thought, *why is this?* I remembered when I used to feel badly about certain kinds of calls, but now it was as if I couldn't care.

I examined my face in the mirror. My eyes seemed dark and hardened. I was only twenty-eight and I felt so much older than that. But those eyes, they'd seen it all: triple shootings, brothers who stabbed sisters, kids drowned in pools, babbling psychotics, teen suicides.... the list was endless.

They call it "burnout," I thought, but I wasn't burned out. I could still do the job; I just couldn't feel the way normal people would feel if they were on these calls. Off-duty I could feel badly about things, not here. How could this have come to be?

What I've seen must have hardened me, but it was more than that. It was as if the whole system and the fire department was pushing me in that direction.

The fire department wants employees to lack emotion, to unquestioningly follow orders. Show no feelings; show no fear; dot your "i's" and cross your "t's"- that's the professional way. Work every call the same with no exceptions. Conform or you'll never go anywhere.

Unfortunately, some calls needed emotions- compassion, tears and, yes- even anger.

But that was the fire department way and, consequently, it tended to smother any kind of creativity you could ever possibly have on the job.

Not that this was wrong; there was no other way to have us do the job. It's how the fire department always was and always would be.

That was true in my case. I remembered back to the first time I got in trouble and the first time the fire department had to remind me that nonconformists would not be accepted here.

I'd been called into the conference room to explain my actions on a call, to explain why I had lost my temper on the scene. I had been "rude" to some other pre-hospital care providers who did a lousy job on a patient before we arrived. It was an eighty year-old lady who lay unconscious, turning as blue as my shirt and nothing was being done. When I vented my anger, I broke the number one rule and used emotion, offending them in the process.

The fact that an eighty-year-old woman almost died due to the negligence of others who knew better was never brought up or even addressed later. I ended up saving her life and getting a disciplinary letter in my file. I pleaded my case but those in the conference room did not even attempt to hear me.

So that was the start: I was being molded into one of them. Those in the conference room had made it clear that they would rather have you mediocre and machine-like as opposed to good and wild.

After that and a few other minor instances, the idea of staying out of trouble began to appeal to me and, little by little, I must have changed, or better yet- conformed.

* * *

Closing my eyes, I imagined the Reverend alive, cooking dinner just two days before Easter. There was a knock at the door. He looks through the peephole, recognizes the young man and methodically unlocks the three locks on his door.

He was not a churchgoer, but a neighborhood boy. They talk about trivialities. He figures he's here for a loan, as he's been there before. The boy has trouble holding a job.

More talk of more trivialities, weather and whatnot. The Reverend goes back to stirring his food and suddenly the boy comes upon him. He feels his strong arm around his neck. He cannot speak or yell. The boy's other hand is hitting him across the face. He can no longer see out of his right eye. The struggle ensues.

The boy's one arm releases its grip and goes away for a minute and then as quickly as it went away, it comes back. What's that in his hand? A knife? No, not you, not now.

He begins to struggle harder, getting some breathing room now. He pleads and screams for help simultaneously.

The hand with the knife moves quickly and then there is

nothing but darkness.

* * *

I continued to look in the mirror. A Reverend had been murdered on Easter weekend and I felt neither anger nor cried any tears.

I wondered what happened to that little boy who grew up in New Jersey, who used to jump in piles of leaves, who wanted to be a professional football player and who was considered so sensitive for his age.

Be professional; join the Fire Department. That's what those in the conference room wanted, and they did an excellent job because I was so impersonal now, so professional, I couldn't even tell you the Reverend's name. Approximately seventy-five-year-old, male and average size was the best I could do.

As I stared in the mirror I felt and watched as the tears rolled down my cheeks. But they were not normal tears, they were bitter tears and not for a poor, old man who'd been murdered like they should have been, but for me and the monster I'd become.

Headhunters

From the day he started he was warned about them. They stopped at nothing to get what they wanted- their justice. Get on their list, make one wrong move and they'd get you; they'd have your head.

"You mean the guys in the white shirts?" he asked naively.

"Ah, some- but mainly the guys in the offices," somebody replied in a whisper.

The years went by like light years in a science fiction movie. He was proud of the patches he wore: the fire department patch on his left arm and the paramedic patch on his right.

He remembered why he had joined the department. What was he- all of nineteen? It had happened so quickly: the park, the kids, the intracoastal. A splash, then another and before he knew it he was carrying the little boy out of the water, slicing up his arm in the process.

Scars, but scars of courage. Something to be proud of. A hero, they called him. What a feeling!

Before that, he'd just been floating through life and careers. At that point he knew what he wanted to be, and because the years had gone by so quickly, the memory was at best sketchy now. A letter of discipline, some time off, a stupid mistake and now, they were after him.

Beware of the Headhunters!

He remembered when he used to laugh at them. Sitting around the coffee table in the morning, they all would joke, but now he was scared.

Seen it all; done it all. His peers thought he was "burned out", that he didn't care.

Golden boy. His shine was tarnished now, and one could worry oneself to death trying to make everything right. But when they were after someone, everything could be right and they'd still find a way to get you. They just bided their time.

Beware of the Headhunters!

More responsibility. At times, he couldn't bear it. Everyone could take their shot: the families would complain about your attitude, the nurses about your treatment, the captains about your duties and the doctors about everything in general. You had no rights; you were always guilty until proven otherwise.

This was all fuel for the fire, the fire the Headhunters had started in order to make him sweat. They didn't care about right or wrong; only their justice mattered.

Paranoia. It had set in. He checked everything twice. He couldn't sleep. Did he fill out those forms right? Was that done? Was this the way it should've gone?

Fifty decisions a day; fifty possible mistakes. Fifty cans of fuel. All he had wanted to do was help people, to get that feeling back he'd had in the park.

Life. What else could he have done? A lawyer, a businessman: would he have succeeded?

Now, he stands alone, wondering about rules and operating procedures because he's on their list. Some say he's one of the best, but that doesn't matter to the Headhunters.

He knows they're close and he's up to two packs a day.

An ulcer at twenty-nine? Old men have those. They have worry lines, too, and so did he. He whispers when he speaks. A sudden move and he spins around. Was that them?

Turning back, he looks deeply into a sunset, lighting up a cigarette and popping a Digel, trying to remember that nineteen-year-old in the park that one fateful day.

Eyes of Innocence

Junior's one-year-old and two months now, or is he one and three? I don't know- time just flies. He's growing right in front of me.

Most of whatever he does, he learns. He can almost talk. I mean he says, "Dight," instead of light and "Tot" instead of hot, but you know what he's saying.

He's a little me and that's what he wants to be. He plays with a bright red toy fire engine and can imitate a siren at times upon request.

I remember I wasn't that happy when I first heard about Junior, but when he was born it was the greatest day in my life.

If only my marriage could have held up better. Oh well separation, in lieu of divorce, seems to be the American Way nowadays.

Every time I leave him I spend the rest of the week thinking about him: his little fingers touching mine, the games we played. I wonder what he's doing or maybe if he's learned something new. And his eyes like two dark computer chips, take it all in, process it, and then he thinks about it and his hands try it, whatever it is.

Eyes of innocence.

"Da-da," he said the other day. And he meant me!

Age has begun to sink in and with it, it's dawned on me that I'm not immortal. Like the patients I treat, someday I will die. But Junior is my next 70 years.

I affect his life in every way. He remembers things we've done, the words I've said. And when I bring him home and lay him down to sleep, kissing him goodnight, I look into those eyes of innocence. He knows nothing yet of fear, hate or even real love.

Those dark brown eyes see everything the same- without evil. And when he tries to look in mine I wonder what he sees: the needless stabbings, the useless shootings, the mutilated bodies, the babbling psychotics- some of the worst moments of humankind?

So when I kiss him goodnight for another week, I close my eyes quickly, hoping the innocence of his eyes will never turn into the eyes of his father.

Zard

When the call came in, it seemed like just your typical "zard run." I figured we'd just go over to that nursing home and pick up the "lizard" and either turf him over to the ambulance, or if it was serious, we'd transport him to the hospital ourselves in the rescue truck. Either way, we'd do it fast.

I hated these "zard runs". We had nicknamed them such since the lizard was one of the oldest living reptile-remnants left over from the dinosaur days. That was typical fire department humor: we made fun of everything and gave everything a another name, even each other. There was Sloth and Axeman, Batman and Joystick, and, of course, me, Brawny-"the quicker- picker- upper."

It was your typical nursing home run by your typical nursing home staff. After waiting five minutes at the back door, an oblivious apathetic nurse waddled over to let us in, saying, "Why are you here?"

"I would guess somebody called us," I said, shaking my head, disgusted with the non-caring, uninformed treatment these places usually gave. The nurse just stared at us as we humped our equipment inside. *Must be one helluva emergency*, I thought.

It took another seven or eight minutes as we followed this oblivious nurse so that she could ask several other oblivious nurses if they'd called us.

They all replied the same. "Huh?...Not me."

What a way to go, I thought. *To die a lizard in a place where no one cares.*

Finally we found the one who called us and she took us to the room. The patient was an eighty-five-year-old male who had fallen five hours earlier. In the meantime he'd not eaten much dinner, seemed like he was out of it and couldn't walk when they tried to take him to the bathroom. We examined his leg; it looked like he'd broken his femur. There was extremity shortening and swelling in the mid-thigh area.

I found out later his name was Arnold King and due to a stroke he couldn't speak coherently. That night he said nothing at all. When I tried to talk to him, it seemed like he was trying to tell me something. He fidgeted with my uniform sleeve, tried to touch my badge.

Most of all, however, he looked sad.

Due to the stench of urine, which was the odor of choice in most nursing homes, and the fact that the patient was obviously unhappy, I told my partner, "Let's get outa here." *I'll get the lizard; you get the paperwork.*

We placed a splint on his leg, so the ride to the hospital was longer than usual. In that time Arnold tried to tell me that something. He pointed and made gestures with his hands. He had some secret.

We dropped him off at the ER and because of another call, I didn't get a chance to check back in on him. I just remembered him touching my badge and those sad deep, ocean blue eyes.

I'd never forget those eyes.

Arnold King's name came up again about four weeks later when I read his obituary in the paper. I remembered the name and the call. His obit was unusually brief, but unlike most lizards in that condition, his funeral was listed the following day at a very nice local funeral parlor.

It seemed crazy, but I figured seeing his name was almost an act of God, so I decided to swing by the funeral the next day. Besides, I just couldn't get those eyes out of my head.

Naturally I was late, arriving after the eulogy. There were only a handful of people paying respects, all old men. Immediately something struck me as funny: there was fire department paraphernalia all around the room, complete with posters, plaques and old-time pictures.

One of the old men approached me. "Did you know Arnie?" he asked.

"Ah," I began. I wasn't sure how to handle this, so I decided to just tell the truth. "Not really, I took him to the hospital once; I work for the Fire Department."

"Really." He nodded his head, thoughtfully. "So did I; so did Arnie. He was my Battalion Chief." He paused. "I should say 'Kingsey'- that's what we called him." He pointed to the rest of the room. "As a matter of fact we all worked at New York Fire Department, you know, up north."

A Chief, I thought. That was his secret; that's what he wanted to say to me. He was remembering.

The old man and I spoke for about 45 minutes before I left to go home. He told me several stories about he and Arnold and then thanked me, saying, "I know old Kingsey would've appreciated a young firefighter comin' to his funeral."

During the drive home I could think of nothing but Arnold King. To think a lizard like that could have been a respected chief in a previous life was unbelievable. A fellow Brother dying alone. He must have outlived his family and wound up with only his fire department buddies to visit and care for him.

At home, I studied my face in the mirror. I saw a young, strong man who'd been wrong.

I've changed lately. I've stopped referring to those calls as "zard runs" and I've stopped calling the patients lizards. It's funny- I'm the first one to have mentioned those nurse's attitudes, but I never noticed I had one as well. Now when I have an elderly patient from a nursing home I listen when they speak and I try to feel when they feel. I'm even trying to work with the nursing homes to improve their treatment, and lately, I never judge someone until I know them.

The other day I again looked in the mirror. I no longer saw a young man, but a more fair one. Because I figure when I'm old and gray and long forgotten, I'd like to think maybe one young firefighter just might attend my funeral to say good-bye to someone he'd never known.